"Written with clarity and a passion earned through his own journey, Fiveson's book offers an integrated approach that can help anyone on a journey of self-discovery."

ALLEN SALKIN,
A REPORTER FOR THE NEW YORK TIMES, VANITY
FAIR, AND LOS ANGELES MAGAZINE.

"In The Mindfulness Experience, executive-life coach and two-time cancer survivor Keith Fiveson delivers a comprehensive guidebook to living a more balanced, sane, and fulfilling life in the face of uncertainty and adversity. Filled with real world insights, quick tips, actions steps, and much needed encouragement, Keith surveys eight key strategies from meditation and exercise, to sleep regulation and relationships, gleaned over his twenty-five years, to help us access the hidden well of wellness deep within us. At a time when there are as many distractions as there are growing concerns to divide our attention, disconnect us from our bodies, and separate us from each other and Spirit, The Mindfulness Experience helps bring us back into connection and coherence as elegantly as a singing bowl."

DR. MILES NEALE,
CONTEMPLATIVE PSYCHOTHERAPIST, AUTHOR OF GRADUAL
AWAKENING, AND ADVANCES IN CONTEMPLATIVE

"During this socially crazy, politically turbulent, Pandemic time, "The Mindfulness Experience" is a much-needed recipe for peace and tranquility. Whether you are stressing under the pressure of the corporate world or trying to manage a family or just feeling something could be better, Keith's 8 Strategies can be utilized by anyone to help create a mindfulness state physically, spiritually, and emotionally. I highly recommend it as it will improve your mind, body, relationships and outlook on the world."

DAVE SHAPIRO,
COO, PREMIER BPO

"The beauty of this book is that it doesn't matter where you live, what your religious or spiritual beliefs are, or your economic or social status. The guidance provided herein applies to all human beings striving to live a more complete and fulfilling life."

ZUBIN KAPADIA,
HEALTHCARE ENTREPRENEUR

"Keith Fiveson's highly engaging book The Mindfulness Experience is a must read for anyone striving for balance, beauty, and good health in their lives and with their family and friends. Keith has managed to combine his extensive business and managerial experience with his deep understanding and study of Eastern traditions including becoming a Yogi. As a result, his book is highly readable and provides cogent advice along, as he puts it, the "8 strategies to live life now": Mind, Body, Spirit, Fuel, Recharge, Environment, Relationships, and Aspirations."

BILL PRICE
LEAD CO-AUTHOR OF *THE BEST SERVICE IS NO SERVICE: LIBERATING YOUR CUSTOMERS FROM CUSTOMER SERVICE, KEEP THEM HAPPY, AND CONTROL COSTS* (WILEY, 2008), LEAD CO-AUTHOR OF *YOUR CUSTOMER RULES! DELIVERING THE ME2B EXPERIENCES THAT TODAY'S CUSTOMERS DEMAND* (WILEY, 2015)

"How we seek happiness and fulfillment in life is a universal pursuit. Keith has composed a priceless smorgasbord of options for anyone to construct their ideal path forward. It will appeal to both newbies and experienced people alike with its inviting tone, authentic nature, and wonderful combination of lived examples and pragmatic guidance. Highly recommend to anyone facing challenges in life and seeking to make meaningful, positive, and lasting changes that will affect themselves, others, and the world around them"

- DANIEL SIEBERG,
CO-FOUNDER, AND CHIEF STORYTELLER, *GOODTRUST*

The Mindfulness Experience

8 STRATEGIES TO LIVE LIFE NOW

FIND BALANCE IN AN UNBALANCED WORLD

KEITH W FIVESON

THE MINDFULNESS EXPERIENCE

Eight Strategies to Live Life Now

For information contact:

Keith Fiveson

http://www.workmindfulness.com

Special thanks to my brother Adam Fiveson for his help with the book cover design and the title of the book

ISBN: 978-1-7370818-0-7 (Ingram Spark)

ISBN: 978-1-7370818-9-0 (KDP)

The Mindfulness Experience

8 STRATEGIES TO LIVE LIFE NOW

FIND BALANCE IN AN UNBALANCED WORLD

KEITH W FIVESON

THE MINDFULNESS EXPERIENCE

Eight Strategies to Live Life Now

Copyright © 2021 by Keith Fiveson

This book is a nonfiction work that draws from life experiences and research to provide the reader with the tools needed to live a healthy, proactive life.

For information contact:

Keith Fiveson

http://www.workmindfulness.com

Special thanks to my brother Adam Fiveson for his help with the book cover design and the title of the book

ISBN: 978-1-7370818-0-7 (Ingram Spark)

ISBN: 978-1-7370818-9-0 (KDP)

Table of Contents

Acknowledgments

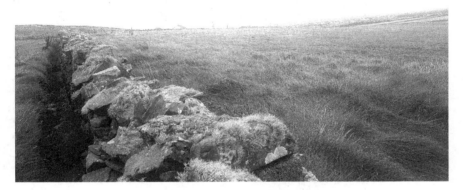

County Claire, Ireland, Ancestry Trip 2019

I HAVE SO much gratitude for this life. It is a distinct privilege to have the chance to write this book as well, as my path in life has not been easy, and frankly, I never thought that I would get to be sixty-five years of age. I've been through a lot.

Yet, my many trials and tribulations have called upon me to seek a more balanced and direct path through the chaos and upheaval. But as my dad would often say, "You live and learn, or you don't live long…"

I owe a huge deal to all the people who helped me write this book. I relied on the wisdom of the ages and today's science data for much of the knowledge and insights that I've outlined in it.

For the past twenty-six years, my wife, Charlotte, has continued to inspire, confound, and challenge me with her love and ability to wake me up. More than anyone, she has called me and challenged me to live a better life, and because of her steadfastness, I have. She is my beloved and my worthy opponent, as she has taught me how to be present in life, challenging me to be the best version of myself.

I'd also like to thank my friends and family (my sons, Justin and Michael; our daughter, Scottie; and our seven grandchildren, Gunnar, Damian, Eliza, Robbie, Lily, Allie, and R. J.). I'd especially like to thank my friend, Shawn, who has taught me how to lighten up, laugh, and venture into the wilds, to enjoy nature and all of its wild glory. And as well, I'd like to thank my friend, Fiona, who has given me her spark of Irish wit and limerick, and Arzanne, who inspired me to find my voice. All my friends and family have inspired me throughout my career and personal life with their insights and humor. I am forever grateful for their lights, for offering me hope and challenges, that I might lift myself and rise to new heights.

Finally, I would like to thank the Veterans Administration (VA) for the benefits I was awarded because I served my country in the US Army. Also, I received the GI Bill, which helped me to go to college. They provided me with the foundation that I've used in this book and throughout my life. For more information, reference the VA Health and Wellness Guidelines link below.[1]

Letter to the reader

The ideas presented throughout this book came to me before and during the Coronavirus pandemic. COVID has rapidly shifted the world's perspectives on life to a more conservative moment-by-moment view of life's preciousness. With millions of people dead, 2020 was not a year when we got what we wanted. It was a year that helped us to appreciate what we have.

Many governments worldwide have mandated facemasks, social distancing, and reduced contact for those deemed at risk. Deaths, job losses, and wild swings in the financial markets have impacted everyone in one form or another. Shaped by COVID, reality has changed for all humans on the planet. Just facing the challenges of everyday life can be maddening. We also had a heatedly contested presidential election in 2020, and it's an understatement to say that what used to be normal has changed. When the pandemic hit, none

---

1   https://www.va.gov/WHOLEHEALTH/docs/10-773_PHI_May2020.pdf

of us were ready or sure how long it would last. Shifts happen, and our world has shifted toward a new normal; it is now in need of an alternative way of life.

At the time I am writing this, over 600,000 have died in the USA, and those numbers continue to rise. The virus has impacted millions around the world. Over the past year, they have restricted people to stay at home. Preventative measures, remaining six feet apart, washing hands, wearing masks, and staying at home have all become part of the new normal. Thousands of people have died in hospitals, and families have suffered. Unemployment has risen, and thousands of businesses have closed. We need to be more mindful. Mindfulness and a focus on ourselves through our breath have never been more critical. Forced to be indoors, more humans have a more refined appreciation for life. We are becoming sapient human beings, growing in our knowledge and connection to what is around us and the world outside. We are mindful of wearing masks and staying healthy in mind, body, and spirit.

Who am I, and why am I writing this book?

I was raised in Brooklyn, New York City. I had it rough as a kid but still loved to play and ride my bike. We played on the streets and in the local parks. Various games occupied us after school and on the weekends.

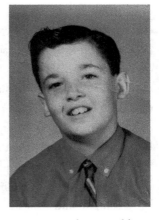

My favorite game, which I was very skilled at, is called "hide-and-seek." I was an expert, knowing how to pick the best spots for hiding in, being quiet, and blending in. I was around eight years old when I learned how to focus on breathing to be quiet and still. Staying perfectly still was a

Me at eight years old, a hide and seeker

discipline. Combined with breath control, it calmed down any movement, and I thought I was invisible and undetectable. Back then, my hide-and-seek strategy worked, and I won so often that people would give up. The same approach was helpful in my home life as well.

My childhood was a bit like living in a war zone. My home was dysfunctional. Mom and Dad were primarily absent from my life. Dad left when I was just a little kid, and Mom drank a lot (she self-medicated with alcohol to ease her pain). I was what we nowadays call a latchkey kid. The only difference was that Mom was home but just not available. Trust was dangerous; hide-and-seek was safer. I was an introvert, submerged my thoughts and feelings, blended in wherever possible, and took an interest in magical things (things believed in but not seen). I took refuge in the solitude of my mind, the popular music of the day, and quiet solitude, often while internally shouting, screaming, and "acting out" some drama, like being a truant, runaway, or delinquent.

It was the '60s, and my family and my world were a complicated mess—alcohol, drugs, gangs, violence—a dangerous place for me. Alan Watts, Ravi Shankar, Maharishi Yogi, the Beatles' music, and the philosophy of Eastern meditators helped me find some peace. I found my breath, body, mind, and spiritual things inspiring. I aspired for a better life and was interested in transcendental meditation, astrology, and the cosmos.

My teens were what you would call troubled. My dad took custody of me when I was thirteen, and it was difficult to leave my mother. I could not adapt to everyday life and first ran away at fifteen. At seventeen, I was a maladaptive teen; I left the comfort of my dad's home in Scarsdale, New York, and found myself on the streets of New York City, homeless. I took refuge at the Salvation Army and found a job washing dishes in Mount Airy, Pennsylvania, before moving to Florida and working at the Boca Raton Hotel and Club. There, I met a group of friends and left for a hippie commune in New Hampshire. I met quite a few beautiful people, and I am still friends with them after forty years. After a year and a half of that, I found my way into the US Army—another communal life, but just more disciplined. At twenty years of age, I dedicated myself to the discipline and education I received from life in the army, and I committed myself to the goal of traveling extensively around the world.

My army experience was a Zen-like existence. I was focused, self-reliant, and learned how to manage my feelings and gain mastery over my perspective by becoming aware of my thoughts and mind. I learned to organize myself, finding structure in the rigorous training I received. This later became the foundation for a successful career in the communications industry.

I was recognized as an achiever and received a top-secret clearance for my work with the Ballistic Missile Defense Communications Activity (BMDCA). Initially stationed in the US—New Jersey, Georgia, Arizona—I was also transferred to Germany. I went to college, learned skills, and paved the way for a profession in telecommunications. Eventually, I received a B.S. in communications and an M.Div. in interfaith studies. I did an executive MBA at Fordham University, while I was working at MCI Telecommunications.

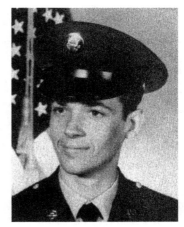

My US Army Photo, 1975

Over the past thirty years, I have received training and certificates, and I have worked as a yoga teacher, massage therapist, interfaith minister, mindfulness teacher, addiction recovery coach, counselor, and executive coach to high-performing professionals, which is what I do now. I worked for Fortune 50 corporations and even had a consulting firm called I.T. Enabled Services Alliance, Inc., during the outsourcing wave. I ultimately retired from Price Waterhouse Coopers, as a management consultant, in 2016.

My career was successful but not without casualties. I had not learned to manage my stress or childhood trauma along the way. I destroyed two marriages, had cancer twice, and suffered from heart issues. Yet, I still found inner inspiration along the way. Through my relationships with my son Justin, my wife of over twenty-six years, my stepchildren Scottie and Mike, and my seven grandchildren, I have found the spirit and aspiration to go forward and continue to try for a better version of myself.

I wrote this book when it became clear that some basic principles had worked and helped me over the years. It's not a perfect world, but we can make it better.

Introduction

YOU ARE THE expert on your own life, values, goals, and priorities. No one will argue with your commitment if you are committed. You are the only one who can know and understand what matters to you. Self-knowledge will help you to live a more mindful and balanced approach to your health and wellness.

The eight strategies in this book will help you create an inside-out and outside-in balance that is perfect for your health and wellness. The self-assessment, mindfulness scripts, and links are designed to show how much more of life's colors we can see when we open our eyes to the world around us.

Being fully aware of your experiences, paying attention to what is happening at the moment, and enhancing it with your awareness is the key to health and wellness. Often, we go through daily life on autopilot, not fully aware of the present. We dwell on the past, plan the future, and get hijacked from paying attention to what is essential at the moment, happening right now. Your body and mind regularly send signals. But if your attention is elsewhere, you don't notice the little things, and what began as a small signal becomes a loud warning.

When you miss the small signal of an early discomfort, a hurt, or a sad feeling, you miss opportunities to make changes before they turn into full-blown pains or anxiety disorders. Being mindful or aware allows you to make conscious, proactive choices about every aspect of your health. Mindfulness connects you to each component of your well-being and your entire self.

Find balance from the inside out—and the outside in

There are many ways to stay healthy and happy. And while it's essential to have an up-to-date care plan for your health, you're the only person who can decide what happens with yourself from inside out or outside in; this includes what goes into your ears, eyes, and mouth so that you can remain focused on staying balanced no matter where life takes you next!

During these days of the pandemic, it is easy to get lost and unbalanced in the world of opinions, news, and compromise. Your outside community of relationships with friends and family and your environment have changed. Now it's more important to have a supportive network of friends and family that serve you, care for you, and hear and recognize you for who you are. For some, their community is close; and for others, it is far away. Your neighborhood is more than where you live, work, and worship. It includes all the people and groups you connect with, who rely on you, and whom you trust. It is the world outside your inner circle. When you balance your internal needs against the outer world, make sure you do so with care and compassion.

The first five strategies look at how to take care of your mind, body, and spirit in order to refuel and recharge yourself through sleep and rest. The following three methods look at balancing your relationships, environment, and aspirations from the outside in. When you combine them, these eight strategies will help you develop your strength and power in the world. Use them as a part of a mindful program of awareness to prevent and treat disease or dis-ease.

Eight strategies for living life now

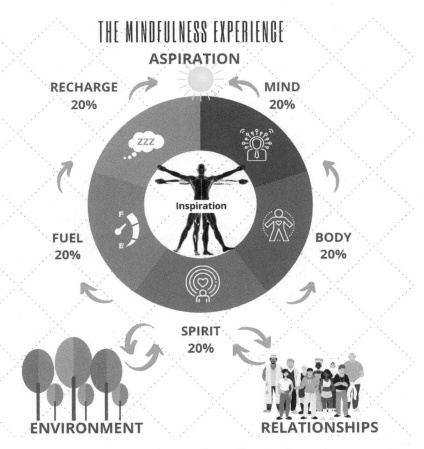

THE MINDFULNESS EXPERIENCE

ASPIRATION

RECHARGE 20%

MIND 20%

FUEL 20%

BODY 20%

Inspiration

SPIRIT 20%

ENVIRONMENT

RELATIONSHIPS

Eight Strategies Visual - From the Inside-out and Outside-in

How you take care of yourself will significantly impact your health and well-being more than the medical care you receive. Each of these eight strategies for finding balance will contribute tremendously to you being balanced and healthy. At the end of each chapter, I will ask you to do a quick assessment of how you rate yourself in each of the areas. I will also ask you to place yourself against where you'd like to be. Consider this to be a "check-in" with your health gaps and a planning tool for taking the first step towards living a healthier life.

Chapter 1: Mind–Strengthen and Focus

How you use your mind is an inside-out strategy. Your mind can affect your body and your perspective on the world. Sometimes your mind runs wild without your awareness. It's like the mind has a mind of its own. Your brain ruminates and thinks about stressful things, and heart rate and blood pressure rise, while breathing becomes shallow. But, when you bring awareness to thoughts, you can direct your mind to lower your blood pressure, control pain and regulate breathing. You will learn to use the connection between your body and mind. Warriors and athletes use the mind's power to visualize a successful mission or event. Mind–body practices tap into the power of the mind to heal and cope.

Chapter 2: Body–Energy and Flexibility

How you use your body, well, that too is an inside-out strategy. When the body feels good your mind feels good too. Exercise gives you energy, strength, and power. Movement can make you more flexible. Regular exercise can lower blood pressure, cholesterol, and help you reduce the risk of heart disease. The heart and lungs are essential organs in your body. You will learn how to leverage your exercise and movement by including walking, gardening, dancing, or lifting weights. It is essential to find what works for you.

Chapter 3: Spirit–Growing and Connecting

Your spirit, or breath, is also an inside-out strategy. A sense of meaning and purpose in life is vital to many people. When things are hard, where do you turn for strength and comfort? Some people turn to spiritual or religious faith. Others find solace in nature, connect with art or music, or prefer quiet time alone.

Chapter 4: Fueling–Eat and Nourish

The "fuel" that you pour into your body is an inside-out strategy. What you eat and drink can nourish your body and mind, do nothing, or destroy your body. You are the gatekeeper of your mouth. In this chapter, we look at how to choose healthy eating habits that fit your lifestyle. Use supplements that support your health goals, and limit alcohol, caffeine, and nicotine. Overall, what you put in your body either gives you power or takes it away. Keep your body and mind adequately fueled.

Chapter 5: Recharge–Sleep and Refresh

When and how you recharge is an inside-out strategy. This chapter looks at sleep and rest as essential ingredients for growing and maintaining your body and mind. Rest gives you peace. Relaxation lowers stress. Activities you enjoy can help you feel recharged. The right balance between exercise and rest improves your health and well-being and keeps you balanced.

Chapter 6: Environment–Physical and Emotional

What does your home or office say about you? This outside-in strategy looks at how your environment can affect your health. It looks at how some settings can give you energy, how others can take it away, and how safety problems like clutter, noise, bad smells, low lighting, or water quality can impact your health. You may be able to change some of these, but not all of them. I give you insights into how to start by paying attention to how your environment influences your life and health. Improve what you can. It's profitable to have a safe, comfortable, and healthy space

Chapter 7: Relationships–Love, Friends, and Marriage

We start with our inner relationship and then move to the outside-in relationships. Be on guard that you don't take on feelings of loneliness, from being alone. Feelings of loneliness can make you sick or keep you sick. You may be alone, yet able to cultivate positive social relationships that are healthy. Having healthy, intimate relationships with friends or a life partner can be a source of strength. It is wise to talk to people who care about you and listen to you. This chapter explores ways to better connect with a community of friends and family.

Chapter 8: Aspiration-Learning and Growing

Aspirations occur when we are needing to find balance or are already well-balanced. No matter where you are in life, your personal and work lives are significant. In this chapter, we look at how you can spend time on areas that generate energy. They affect not only your happiness but also your health. What inspires and gives you power on the inside? Your ability to empower yourself will enable you to aspire for more on the outside. What are the best ways of spending my available energy every day? Do things give me strength and power, or do they take it away? Who, what, or where makes me weak and tired? Do I do the things that matter most to me?

Using this book and the eight strategies outlined will help balance your inner world and develop insights. With insight, we can care for our minds, bodies, and spirits with fuel (food, drink) and recharge with some sleep—and thus find balance in an unbalanced world. These strategies show us how to balance our inner world, integrate and strengthen our resilience and connections, and inspire our aspirational lives.

With aspiration, our outer-world strategies focus on relationships and our immediate environments. When we have a healthy inner world, we can better balance our external world energies, inspire others in our everyday environments, and aspire to even higher levels of realization.

By integrating the inner and outer worlds, we can develop our ability to inspire, aspire, and envision possibilities in the world. This book will help you cope with this crazy world and rise above it by energizing, empowering, and inspiring changes so you can live a more powerful life.

I hope this book will provide you with the insight and knowledge to do just that!

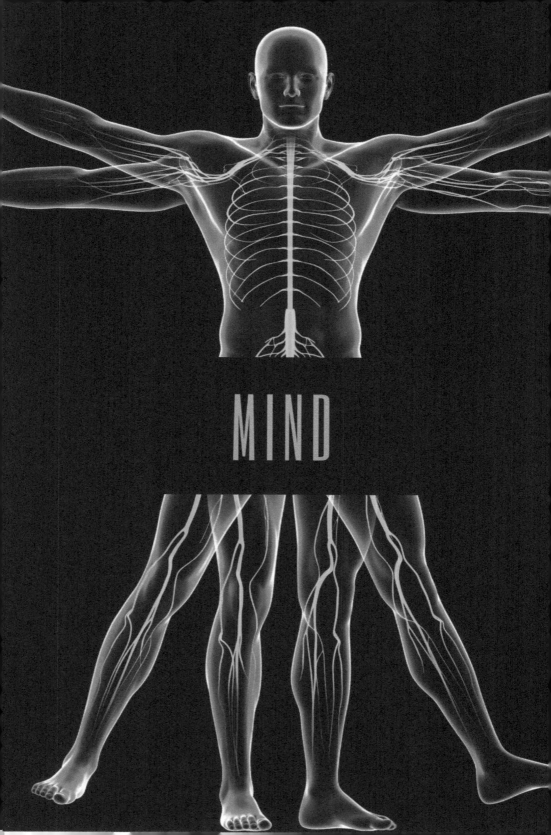

Chapter 1

MIND

Strengthen and Focus

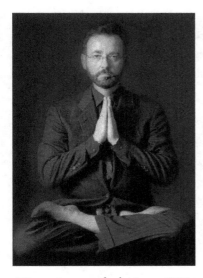

Promoting yoga for business, 1995

IN THIS CHAPTER we look at the nature of mind. We ask, what does it mean to "be in our right minds?" That phrase describes calm, reasonable, and sane people who don't climb into lion enclosures at the zoo or put themselves or others in harm's way. When people are in their right minds, they make rational decisions and benefit themselves and others. They seek to work in understandable ways. They don't drive their cars off of cliffs or into snowbanks. You may suspect you are not in your right mind if you come home from an animal shelter with seven dogs or cats.

Our minds affect our bodies, spirits, and ability to metabolize food, and even our sleep, rest, and recharge patterns. If you let your mind meander without taking hold of it, it can be a terrible meaning-making machine. We must learn how to manage and control our senses because they can unleash an internal chemical storm that creates stress and increases our heart rate and blood pressure. This chapter looks at how to use our mind's power to breathe, focus, gain awareness of our bodies, and lower our blood pressure. We learn how we can even manage and control pain by focusing our minds.

The US Marine Corps knows how to use the mind's power to visualize successful missions or events. Professional athletes and regular people train with mind–body techniques to tap into powerful breathing and visualization practices to heal and cope with stress and trauma. There is nothing on Earth that is more powerful—or destructive—than the power of the mind. It should carry a warning label! We must use it with care and not waste it on senseless activities, numb it, or dumb it down. Our minds have the power to heal and the power to destroy.

Accessing Energy, Information, and Flow

What is mindfulness?

In his book, **The Mindful Brain: Reflection and Attunement in the Cultivation of Well-Being**, Daniel J. Siegel, Director of the Mindsight Institute, Co-Director of the UCLA Mindful Awareness Research Center, and the author of several books, writes:

> *"Mindfulness in its most general sense is about waking up from a life on automatic and being sensitive to novelty in our everyday experiences. With mindful awareness, the flow of energy and information that is our mind enters our conscious attention and we can both appreciate its contents and come to regulate its flow in a new way. Mindful awareness, as we will see, actually involves more than just simply being aware: It involves being aware of aspects of the mind itself. Instead of being on automatic and mindless, mindfulness helps us awaken, and by reflecting on the mind we are enabled to make choices and thus change becomes possible."* [2]

Dr. Siegel's definition of mindfulness helps us realize that everyone can be aware, awake, and alive to what is going on around them. Everyone has the power to change their experiences and perspectives and to change their

---

2   Daniel J. Siegel, *The Mindful Brain: Reflection and Attunement in the Cultivation of Wellbeing*, (W.W. Norton & Company April 1, 2007)

energies and the world around them. Mindfulness is like a superpower inside of us. But we must plug it in and switch it on!

We human beings have practiced mindfulness for over 3,500 years, from before the time of the Buddha. In the Vedas, around 1500 BCE, we read about meditation as a spiritual path, concentration exercise, and religious practice. Meditation has a long tradition in Hinduism, Buddhism, Christianity, and other religious practices over the centuries. The Upanishad Hindu texts discuss meditation to remove ignorance and gain knowledge and oneness. But what does this mean exactly? In recent years, scientific evidence has proven that mindfulness is beneficial for managing stress and trauma. We can use it to create a sense of integrity (oneness) while gaining a deeper awareness of what we have and need to do with our lives from inspirational and aspirational perspectives.

These types of aspirational practices can help individuals work with each other on improving conditions worldwide. More and more people continue to be impacted by viruses and sickness and experience more trauma. The Coronavirus Pandemic and increasing concerns about violence, social, political, and economic divides have created a sense of instability and a frantic, disconnected, and unbalanced population. People's interdependencies with each other, nature, communities, and their surroundings have never been more apparent. Finding a sense of balance in an unbalanced world has never been more critical.

Globally, our society, along with our planet, is in trouble. We cannot divorce ourselves from our connections to the earth that sustains us and our humanity. Through mindfulness practice, we connect to our oneness, our fundamental human nature. By allowing fresh air to feed our breath and circulate oxygen throughout our bodies, we notice the inflow/outflow and our bodies sitting on the earth, and we see the water and blood moving throughout our bodies. By connecting to our oneness, we can feel the life-giving force moving within us and find inspiration within and aspiration in the world.

Many people want to practice mindfulness because they think it offers a solution to all their problems. Mindfulness can deal with many of the adverse conditions we face in life—physical issues (such as chronic pain), psychological distress, depression, or anxiety. But it is also beneficial if we want to increase our concentration, creativity, and productivity, or be in harmony and balance with ourselves as we connect with the world.

What are the benefits of mindfulness?

- Improves brain function—improves executive functioning, structural changes, and brain processes; promotes blood circulation; possibly prevents dementia and increases neurogenesis (the brain's capacity to generate new brain cells).

- Improves general health—increases the ability to manage pain; enables more control of symptoms; helps us face disease; confers a metabolic benefit; corrects hormonal changes, changes in function, and aids genetic repair.

- Improves mental health—prevents relapse of depression; lessens anxiety, panic disorder, stress, and improves emotion regulation; promotes emotional intelligence; improves sleep quality; decreases personality disorders and addictions.

- Improves the spiritual sphere—increases inner peace, perceptions, tolerance, and our understanding of others and ourselves.

- Improves your performance—in sports, studies, work, and communicating with others.

Mindfulness in the West

Meditation is associated with the East. The West opened up to meditation as a contemplation practice with the advent of mindfulness. Mindfulness today is free from the spirituality that accompanies religious devotion.

Maharishi Mahesh Yogi introduced Transcendental Meditation to California in the late 1950s. It quickly became a trend in the 1960s, popularized by the Beatles and '60s culture. I grew up in that time, and it profoundly impacted me as a young teenager. Today, it has again caught the imagination of many. Much of it is neuroscience proving that meditation has a direct beneficial impact on the mind and body, with or without a spiritual component. The scientific evidence of its benefits has caused mainstream media to take notice. Dr. Herbert

Benson, a mind/body professor of medicine at Harvard Medical School, conducted the first research on mindfulness meditation. His results created quite a stir, as Dr. Benson noticed how mindfulness meditation produced a response that countered stress. Dr. Benson's book, *The Relaxation Response* became a bestseller and the term "relaxation response" was a term that was often used.[3]

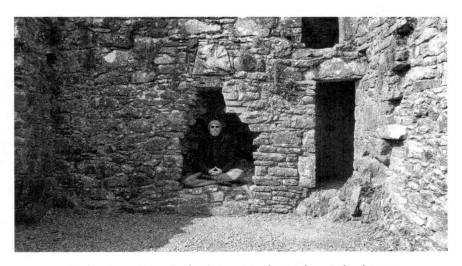

Meditating at Trim Castle, County Meath, Northern Ireland, 2019

The significant differences between "mindfulness" and "meditation" are more around form and formality. Mindfulness looks to strengthen the awareness of your awareness of the present moment, wherever you are. Whereas meditation is about setting aside time for visualization, breath awareness, mantras, or guided practice. Mindfulness focuses your attention on your breath, body, and sense impressions. It helps to emotionally regulate stressful conditions occurring in the sympathetic nervous system through noticing and being present with whatever you're doing. When you are actively mindful of your breath and body, you see the world around you, your thoughts, feelings, behaviors, movements, and the effect you have on those around you.

---

3   Dr. Herbert Benson, *The Relaxation Response* (William Morrow Paperbacks 1975)

How Is Mindfulness Practiced?

We often think of mindfulness as a series of exercises that aim at relaxation. In reality, it is the practice of training the mind to pay attention. Peace is nothing but a consequence or a pleasant side effect.

If you are approaching mindfulness for the first time, start gradually, with small sessions lasting five to ten minutes, twice a day. Increase the number of minutes, little by little, in five-minute increments if comfortable. A steady practice incorporates twenty to thirty minutes or more, depending on your motivation and the time available. The ideal is twenty minutes, twice a day. The best position is seated, but you can lie down, so long as you don't go to sleep. You can practice with your eyes open, tilted down, and with a soft gaze. Closing your eyes allows you to focus on your breath, senses, thoughts, and emotions. Should you start to get sleepy, open your eyes wide, keep them open or close them again after a while.

This practice helps us gain insight into our bodies, using the breath as a point of awareness or "anchor." Other anchors are possible, such as the body—skin sensation, sound, smell, taste in the mouth—emotion, thought, and visual elements such as a candle or some other object.

How to start the practice of mindfulness

Before attempting to do anything, it is essential to understand that mindfulness is not a game. You don't need to evaluate a session every time you practice; there is no right or wrong way. Instead, look at every time you practice as an opportunity to focus your mind on your breath, body, or another anchor of awareness intentionally. Practicing awareness is the goal. Bring your mindful awareness back to the point of focus again and again. Think of it as a mental workout. When you get off track and notice it, return to the end of awareness. Doing this is the "practice" of mindfulness.

For example, if you use your breath as your anchor, your goal is not to stay focused on the breath for an extended period. Instead, it is to know what it means to bring attention to the breath. These are two distinctly different things. When your mind wanders, repeatedly return it to your breath. If you focus on the sensations in your body, you know to what extent your mind wanders. Keep returning your awareness to your body's feelings of warmth, coolness, heaviness, lightness, etc. These mindfulness practices converge into a single goal: learning to return to your chosen focus for the moment, with compassion, without judgment, again and again. Learning to develop your sense of awareness without judgment is the practice. You reinforce it again and again.

Everyone's mind wanders away from their intended focus, even people who have been meditating for a long time. Our minds continue walking, jumping from one thing to another. That is what brains do. Our minds look for problems to solve and wander off to find them. The central point of mindfulness is to train our minds to focus on specific points of choice. We give the mind something to do, and as we practice more and more, the entire process becomes a habit, which strengthens our mental focus. With ongoing practice, we develop self-compassion, attention to our present feelings, and a better understanding of forgiveness for ourselves when we go off course.

We develop compassion for ourselves and others by using the same spirit of forgiveness we may give to a child and thus find ourselves in service to others. Self-care and compassion for others provide the most incredible benefits when blending mindfulness with a loving-kindness practice. A loving-kindness technique involves conscious awareness of our intentions by incorporating the ongoing recitation of affirmations. See the Appendix for the complete Loving-Kindness practice and other mindfulness meditations. You can check out the links as well for audio-guided reflections.

Let's Learn to Practice

Here are three primary steps that every practitioner needs to adopt for a more balanced life by using this foundational practice.

1. Write your goals

Goals involve planning. When we do that, we envision the series of steps needed to accomplish our goals. It is not enough to say that we are doing something. We must know the why and how; we must visualize and outline the steps necessary. Not having a goal in mind is like trying to get directions from a map without knowing your destination. So, to practice mindfulness, it is necessary to set your intention right before you practice. Are your intentions for your benefit or the benefit of others? Intentions fuel the movement of energy. "How can I be of the most significant help to myself and others?" You don't need to have the answers; you just have to know your goal and intention.

It is helpful to write your goals because writing them makes them real. I use my mobile phone because my hopes and dreams are often on the fly. Usually, I will write easy-to-achieve, short-term goals and make them visible by looking at my intentions every day. I have used Post-it notes and placed them on the bathroom mirror, the door, or the computer screen. Some of them are simple reminders, like "Breathe" or "Slow down."

2. Start with short periods

The best way to practice mindfulness is simply to start! I often say that it takes twenty-one days to make a habit and three days to break it. Procrastination is the biggest enemy. Suppose you wait until you find the "perfect moment"—it will never come! So, my advice is not to wait. Start now, as soon as you can, as time is your most precious commodity. I mean now. Don't waste time. Invest in yourself right now. Take a breath and feel the air on your inhalation, fill your lungs, and if you don't feel it in your belly, take a deeper breath. Do this for ten breaths.

Next, find a quiet place where you can sit for a few minutes without being disturbed. Close your eyes and start following your breath. Observe how your lungs expand with each inhalation and how they relax during exhalation. As your body relaxes, notice how your breath becomes graceful and how the in-breath and the out-breath start to merge. Notice the space between the in- and out-breaths. Notice the rise and fall of your chest and belly, like the movement of waves in an ocean. Feel the coolness of your breath during inhalation and its warmth during exhalation. Feel any other sensations in your body. When your mind wanders, simply and compassionately, return to the noticing, sharpening your focus and then loosening it like waves, in and out. When a distraction comes, watch it consciously. Then let it slip away without holding on to it. Bring your awareness gently back to your breath.

Start with a session of about ten minutes and then progress to about twenty minutes or more. Early in the morning is the best time, which may be challenging. It becomes more comfortable and automatic with practice, as you keep your mind steady in the present moment.

3. Journaling as a form of mindfulness

Writing is not just an art form; it can also become an essential technique for working with your mind and reprogramming and balancing your subconscious to help you achieve your goals. It takes only five to ten minutes a day and is invaluable.

Set intentions and write out a series of specific statements. What are your hopes, dreams, and aspirations? What inspires your body, mind, and spirit? Is it food, people, or things? Look at your story with hindsight, insight, and foresight.

Repeatedly writing and reading these statements helps your mind move. Your subconscious brain actualizes the intentions as a habit and a way of being. You are the master of your fate, the programmer of your mind.

Try this for twenty-one days and see yourself acting differently with no conscious effort. Start with these three quick steps and try to incorporate them into your daily practice.

Twelve Mindfulness Exercises for Your Mind

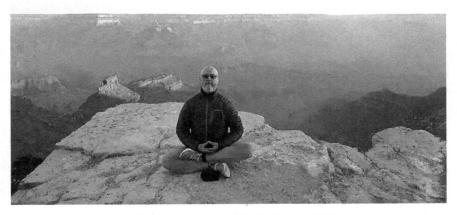

Meditating at sunrise, Grand Canyon, 2016

Often, many of us do not have the time to include a solid mindfulness practice into our morning routine. A typical day already starts early in the morning: alarm, coffee, shower, clothes (dressing for success or hanging out on Zoom) and continues until the evening. Our day goes by quickly at work. Maybe it also involves friends, kids, family pickups, homeschool, check-ups, fast dinners, reading, and television before it's time for bed. Many of us wonder what it's all about and feel a bit unsatisfied with life. We feel moody, perhaps thinking that something is missing. What is it?

Many people live lives of quiet desperation in a concrete jungle, restricted, and far removed from a relationship with nature and themselves. It is increasingly harder to navigate the world outside ourselves when we are just doing our best to get by, especially given the pandemic and trying to stay alive. Many are so busy doing their best to focus on their net worth that they have no time to cultivate their self-worth.

Today's world is about survival, and many people's minds mull over the day's latest news story and traumatic events. Our emotions and thoughts intertwine; we become confused, even depressed about what we can or can't do about it all. We cannot find a logical thread that allows us to feel pleasant, physically or mentally, so we get stressed, anxious, disconnected from ourselves, and disembodied. Often, we can't take five minutes to sit and relax with a loved one or friends and enjoy some fresh air or a park, trees, and nature.

Mindfulness is fundamental to our psychophysical and psychosocial well-being. Like connecting our cell phones with an external cell tower to get a clear GPS signal, it is essential to navigate life and relationships and cultivate our minds.

Twelve tips for cultivating mental muscles

We need to get up a little earlier every day and take time for ourselves at the beginning of the day before we do anything. Early morning is the time to clear our minds and strengthen our inner GPS for connecting with inner calm during a hectic day.

Here are some tips you can use formally when you first wake up or in the evening before getting ready to sleep. Otherwise, you can use them informally during the day, while waiting on hold, or in a line. You can use these tips to sleep better and awaken feeling rested as well. Either way, apply effort, focus, and concentration, with loving-kindness, to make the changes you wish to see.

1. Conscious breathing

You can practice this exercise while standing or sitting anywhere, really, and at any time. All you do is stay still and concentrate on your breathing for one minute or more. It becomes a habit after a while. Just inhale through your nose, filling up your lungs and belly. Exhale slowly through your mouth, as if you are blowing bubbles into a straw. Your inhalation should last about six seconds. Your exhalation through your mouth should last about twelve seconds. Continue this cycle of breathing for ten rounds. Breathing this way activates the parasympathetic side of your autonomic nervous system and helps you rest, digest, and calm your body.

If you think you cannot meditate, know that you are already halfway there with this exercise! If you feel better, relaxed, calm, and charged, escalate the time from one to five minutes, and you will benefit from the long-term effects of this calming practice. Feel the sensations of the breath flowing in and out of your body. Notice the feeling of the air in your nostrils, chest, and belly.

2. Open awareness and observation

This mindfulness exercise is simple but incredibly powerful. It connects you with the beauty of the natural environment. You can easily miss the world when you are in the car or running for a train or bus.

Choose a natural object within the environment surrounding you—a flower, an insect, clouds, or the moon—and concentrate on watching it for a minute or two. Do nothing but watch.

Look at it with curiosity, as if you are looking at it for the first time. Visually explore every aspect of its form and let your focus be wrapped up in it. Allow yourself to connect with its energy and purpose in nature. Relax in harmony with it for as long as your concentration allows.

3. Awareness of awareness

Awareness is at the heart of mindfulness exercises, and this one cultivates your understanding and appreciation of simple daily activities. If you consistently practice it, you will strengthen your mind and focus.

Think of something that happens to you every day more than once, something you take for granted, like opening a door. When you touch the handle to open the door, stop for a moment, and be aware of where you are, how you feel at that moment, and where the door will lead you. Alternatively, you could think of when you turn on your computer to work. Take a moment to appreciate the hands that allow you to perform this process and the brain that understands how to use your device.

You can also do this with your thoughts. Whenever a negative thought comes into your mind, stop for a moment. Label the idea as useless or unproductive and release the negativity. Likewise, whenever you smell food in your home or on the street, take some time to appreciate how lucky you are that you can smell, taste, and enjoy nutritious food with your family and friends.

In this practice, you choose a contact point that inspires you, and instead of automatically going about your day, stop and enjoy whatever it is. Stop and cultivate a proactive awareness of what you are doing and take a moment to be grateful for how it is a part of your life.

4. Listening

My grandmother used to tell me, "God gave us two ears and one mouth; we should listen twice as much as we speak." So, how do we open our ears without judgment? Our past experiences influence what we hear and interpret. It's pretty natural to judge. When we listen with awareness, we are able to be more open, to discern and integrate our experiences. Awareness allows us to listen without preconceptions. Ask yourself, "What is being said, and am I listening?" or "Can I hear the words without moving into emotion?" Focus on your mindful breathing techniques to help your awareness, which will happen with more practice.

For example, focus on a piece of music. Pick a song from your music library or the radio. Practice listening without judgment by closing your eyes and listening to the notes, instruments, and beats without judging them. Can you immerse yourself in the music and allow yourself to explore every aspect? Even if the music is not to your liking at first, can you label your feelings, let go of your dislikes, and enjoy the rhythm, words, or some other aspect of it with awareness? Listen to what others are saying without judgment, and while you may not like them, the tone, or the conversation, you can still be present to the feelings that are arising and find something you can accept.

5. Being present in the moment

Every day we need to do simple tasks that might seem like routine chores, such as washing the dishes. Instead of washing quickly and anxiously to finish as soon as possible, take a moment and pause. Enjoy the moment even if it is an unpleasant task like cleaning the house. It can be an opportunity.

For example, while cleaning the house, pay attention to every detail. Create an unfamiliar experience by noticing every single aspect of your actions. Feel the movement when you sweep the floor, feel the muscles used to move the dishes from the sink to the cupboard, invent a more creative and efficient way to clean the windows.

The idea is to focus on your creativity and discover new experiences in your routine tasks. Instead of continually thinking about ending your job quickly, be aware of each step and completely immerse yourself in it. Treat the activity or task like a dance. Ensure that your body, mind, and spirit come together and have fun while doing your household chores!

An old Zen saying says, "Before enlightenment, chop wood, carry water. After enlightenment, chop wood, carry water." By being in the moment, you no longer feel compelled to watch the clock. Whatever your work might be, bring all of yourself to it. If you are fully present, you may find that your labor is no longer a burden. We may not always be able to control the circumstances we are in or have a lot of say over what needs must get done on any given day. Nonetheless, doing your best at all times will lead to developing good habits and practices which can help you with difficult days when things seem overwhelming.

6. Appreciation

A simple rule to follow in life is to appreciate everything you wish to enjoy and watch it appreciate! Where focus goes, energy flows! Watch your life multiply with this simple exercise. Finish your day by appreciating five things you rarely notice. They can be objects or people—you choose. I use my phone to jot down notes, but you can also use a notepad to write the five things at the end of the day.

The point of this exercise is to experience gratitude for and appreciation of seemingly insignificant things in life. These things sustain our existence, but we often take them for granted. More people are practicing this simple but effective exercise during the COVID pandemic. It is about being happy with what we have rather than merely running after the things we want.

What have we been happy about? You can be pleased about electricity, the mail carrier delivering mail to us every day, or the clothes that keep us warm in winter and offer us freshness in summer. How about our noses that let us smell flowers and the fragrance of freshly baked bread or our ears that allow us to hear bird calls, and so on?

Do you know how these things work? Have you ever stopped to think about how these things benefit your life and the lives of others? Have you ever thought about how your life would be without these things? Just think about how it all works, that somehow through this interconnected web of commerce and distribution, we receive goods, services, and sustenance to survive and thrive. That's a lot to be grateful for, isn't it?

7. Conscious eating

Even lunch or dinner can provide opportune moments for mindfulness exercises. Pay attention to the sensory experiences—consistency, taste, smell—aesthetics, and the sounds you make when you eat.

Savoring food while I eat is one of my favorite activities. It allows me to enjoy every bite, slow down to sense my body digesting it, and eat less. When I am consciously eating, I am not just shoveling food into my belly.

8. Awareness of pause

Between the inhalation and exhalation of your breath, there is a pause. Between each raindrop, there is a space. There are spaces and pauses in everything in life. It's beneficial to find that space in our lives, at work, during breaks, even while walking from one room and entering another. To be present, we have to be aware of our activities and the spaces between the activities.

When there is a break, spend a few seconds away from your desk and look out the window. Use this awareness of a pause and give yourself the gift of recognizing that you are active. Be aware of your body, your life, and your productivity.

There are enough minutes in the day, spaces between those minutes, and spaces between your breaths to be mindful of the gifts in your life.

9. Oxygen-sensory therapy

Bring your attention to your sensations. Pay attention to the feeling of the air on your skin for ten to sixty seconds. This mindfulness exercise works better when you are wearing a short-sleeved shirt, shorts, or sandals, so your skin is exposed to the atmosphere.

10. Sensory body scan

Scan your body from head to toe for any feelings of discomfort or tension. Focus on any sensations—cool, warmth, pressure, and comfort—or any area harboring pain or discomfort. Just be aware of them, label them, and bring an attitude of care, compassion, and awareness without judgment.

11. Acting consciously

Practicing mindfulness requires us to be aware of our awareness. We make a conscious choice to recognize and choose our actions. So, practice mindfulness with daily activity, something habitual you usually do on autopilot. Do it consciously instead. For example, practice mindful awareness while making coffee, breakfast, driving, or walking to work. See if you can look at these activities a bit differently, with fresh eyes.

12. Be mindful, without losing your mind

Just practice, as best as you can, without judgment. Use these exercises when you don't feel comfortable or don't have the time to sit down for any length of time regularly. You don't have to lose your mind because you can practice wherever you are.

Write these exercises on an index card or your phone, and do them to your best ability, one breath at a time, one day at a time.

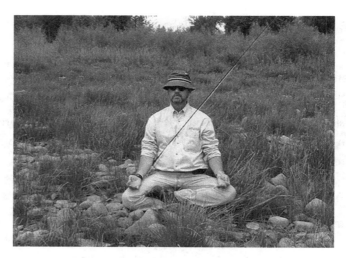

In Missoula, Montana, Fly Fishing, 2011

Mindful Tips

The practice of mindfulness requires that you continue to practice, day after day, moment by moment, wherever you are.

Start slowly and work your way up to more extended sessions. With it, you can let go of the past, move more and more into the present, and not be afraid of future events. By rooting the mind in the present moment, you can face life's challenges more clearly, with an assertive and calm perspective on life.

With more and more practice, you can develop a fully conscious mentality that frees you from imprisonment by useless and self-limiting thought patterns. You can be more mindfully present and focus on positive emotions. Your compassion for and understanding of yourself and others will increase.

How do you rate yourself?

Mind: *Strengthen and Focus*

Tapping into the power of your mind can help you to heal and manage discomfort. By using the breath and body scanning techniques, you can recognize, accept, investigate, and accept your situation or change the outcome.

How do you rate yourself on a scale of 1 (low) to 5 (high)?

Where are you?

1	2	3	4	5

Where do you want to be?

1	2	3	4	5

Why did you choose this number?

_____

_____

_____

What changes could you make to help you get there?

_____

_____

_____

Source: Personal Health Inventory –

Veterans Affairs. https://www.va.gov/WHOLEHEALTH/docs/10-773_PHI_May2020.pdf

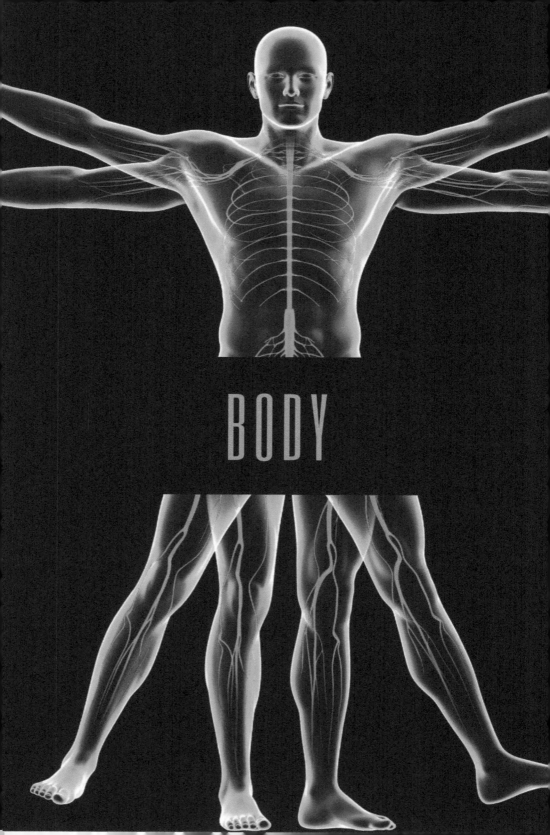

BODY

Chapter 2

BODY

Energy and Flexibility

On Pilgrimage, Thuparama Seya, Sri Lanka 2019

THIS CHAPTER EXPLORES the body and how exercise offers us more energy and access to information and strength when we need it to face the day. We look at how a simple movement can make us more flexible in body and mind. Regular exercise can lower blood pressure and cholesterol and reduce the risk of heart disease. We can exercise, move, stretch, walk, garden, dance, or lift weights; all of these activities are good options. Whatever works for you. If you don't move it, you lose it. Add some visualization techniques, and you will also improve performance, resilience, and overall vigor.

Health and wellness require us to be physically active, maintain sound nutrition, incorporate stress-relief techniques, and maintain a healthy lifestyle. A healthy lifestyle is what keeps us young, more than any beauty product or miracle cure. Regular physical activity in moderation allows us to remain healthy and efficient longer. It delays the degeneration of muscles, joints, and organic structures. Being physically active makes us more present in our bodies and promotes health. It allows us to focus on what generates better experiences for our general health and well-being.

When we are physically active, the whole body benefits, and the neurological effects help increase strength and vitality to balance the body, speech, and mind. There are other proven benefits too.

- We strengthen muscles and joints, improve our posture, and increase resistance to daily fatigue. Abdominal and dorsal muscles get into shape and remove the risk of pathologies in our vertebra (hernias).

- We optimize our metabolism and improve the ratio between our fat mass and lean body mass. We also regulate hunger, and our blood chemistry parameters rebalance themselves.

- We increase our respiratory system's capacity and elasticity, even at rest, due to the increased demand for oxygenation, which the pulmonary alveoli require during exercise.

- We improve the contractile capacity of the heart and its coronary blood supply. At rest, a sports competitor has a lower heart rate than a sedentary person, is less subject to pressure fluctuations, and is more elastic and efficient.

- We fight mood disorders. Physical activity is also beneficial for the psyche and helps fight disorders such as anxiety and depression. Physical activity contributes to the release of two essential types of neurotransmitters: acetylcholine and endorphins. These molecules produce the sensations of analgesia and well-being, so they are known as "happiness hormones."

- Physical exercise also helps us avoid the risk of conditions typical of a sedentary lifestyle: obesity, diabetes, hypertension, and all the pathologies related to the cardiovascular system, including heart attacks, one of the most common causes of death in the Western world.

Research confirms that "a healthy mind in a healthy body" requires that we are mindful of exercising for better memory. A study by the *Journal of the International Neuropsychological Society* on the elderly offers data to show that moderate and regular physical activity can increase the hippocampus's volume and protect against age-related memory decline. The study focuses on both impromptu and intense exercise. Researchers from the University of Maryland used a functional MRI and measured the brain activity of healthy people aged fifty-five to eighty-five. [4]

The volunteers were asked to remember a series of famous and infamous names. Doing this activates a neural network related to semantic memory, which is known to deteriorate over time. The ongoing measurements were carried out both thirty minutes after a moderately intense exercise session on an exercise bike and on a rest day. Examination of the brain activity in four areas of the cortex, including the hippocampus, which is first attacked by Alzheimer's, revealed the volume of the hippocampus increases after physical exercise. People remember, think better, and have better cognition. In *Science Daily*, the study's lead author, Carson Smith, said, "As a muscle adapts to repeated use, individual exercise sessions can modify cognitive neural networks leading to more efficient access to memories." [5]

Better Flexibility is a Must

Body mindfulness is a whole-body experience. It is fundamental for the survival of all people and animals in this world. Whether you practice sports at a competitive level or just need to reach a pot or pan in the kitchen, you need to

---

4   www.sciencedaily.com/releases/2019/04/190425104310.htm.

5   Science Daily, April 25, 2019, www.sciencedaily.com/releases/2019/04/190425104310.htm.

know your flexibility limits and abilities. For those who participate in athletic activities or artistic gymnastics as part of their lives, flexibility is an essential part of their practice. A relaxed person uses the maximum joint width and coordinates their body's functions, joints, muscles, tendons, and ligaments.

Flexibility decreases with increased age. Infants and children are much more flexible than adults. Think about how a baby can bring their foot up to their mouth. Putting your foot in your mouth (literally) is not a simple thing for any adult who is not a contortionist or fully-fledged yogi.

While I can no longer put my feet in my mouth like a child, I sometimes say inappropriate things. For those times and others, I can say that yoga has been an essential part of my mental and physical health and wellness. Stretching and mobility can be trained over time and maintained with daily physical activity. Dedicating myself to my daily workouts, stretching, and back extensions is an essential part of a daily routine. An ongoing yoga stretch practice at the beginning or end of a training session allows my muscles to relax and ensures increased flexibility.

There are active and passive movements to increase flexibility. For active movements, we lengthen the muscles of a body part with no help. With passive stretches we may look to yoga or Pilates (a physical fitness system developed in the early twentieth century by Joseph Pilates) and incorporate passive movement stretches with help of a person, or strap, or even our own legs, to stretch and move mindfully beyond what we can do alone. It is critically important to work with a skilled trainer or movement specialist with passive activities to not overstretch.

It's important to remember:

- With or without more vigorous exercises, stretching must be done progressively, and it's best when the muscles are well warmed up.
- Always respect the physiological limits of your joints.

If you've lived a sedentary lifestyle or have traumas or individual anatomical issues that negatively affect your flexibility, do not push it. Respect the limits of your abilities to stretch, and only go as far as your edge.

How to do physical activity

Everything takes time to build, one day to the next, and when you start, it is necessary to expand your edge slowly, day by day, week after week. Do not try too hard. Don't strain your heart, muscles, or spine with ongoing prolonged exercises, which is a counterproductive mistake that many newcomers or the overly enthused make.

When you stretch and move, you are often covering new terrain, as you may be more accustomed to modern-day comforts (the car, the elevator, the subway). It's better to start with a bit of physical movement: a few flights of stairs or a short walk. Get up from your desk every twenty minutes and take a walk.

Check out the Pomodoro Technique.

There are six steps in the original technique:

1. Decide on the task to be done
2. Set the Pomodoro timer (traditionally to twenty-five minutes)
3. Work on the task
4. End your work when the timer rings and put a checkmark on a piece of paper.
5. If you have fewer than four checkmarks, take a short break (three to five minutes) and then return to step two; otherwise, continue to step six.
6. After four Pomodoros, take a more extended break (fifteen to thirty minutes), reset your checkmark count to zero, and then return to step one.

You can take a stretch and reboot your body and mind.

Exercise helps you to relieve the tension accumulating in your body throughout the day. It allows you to restore and renew your spirits, flood your body with endorphins and serotonin, and stimulate the parasympathetic nervous system. Get up and move when you feel tired.

I have found that doing a minimum amount of stretching every day is superb for my overall health and wellness. But how and when do we try stretching our bodies? What types of stretches should we do as a minimum?

Stretching needs to be a part of our daily routines, but always done mindfully before or after physical exercise. You don't have to do a lot, but make sure you do it to open your body. David Behm, of the School of Human Kinetics and Recreation at the University of Newfoundland Memorial in Canada, conducted a study in stretching sessions with adults over thirty years of age. Here are some results.

There is both dynamic and static stretching. Dynamic stretches are active movements that cause your muscles to stretch, but the stretch is not held in the end position. It allows us to go through a range of motion, somewhat similar to the regular activities or sports we may do during a typical day. Static stretching requires us to hold a stretch for a while without movement, usually only at the end range of a muscle. It offers improvement of the range of motion and movement with a reduced risk of injury. So, let's run through these differences and how you might incorporate them into your daily life.

Stretch—if in doubt, stretch

Static stretching is not as easy as doing nothing because the stretch can be pretty dramatic. Static stretching is like a yin style of yoga, where we hold a pose for a while, and we ask our bodies to relax.

A prolonged stretching session is excellent for getting the kinks and knots out of your body. You can do dynamic stretching to warm up for an activity and then static stretching to come down and relax after the workout. You will find this is especially helpful for you first thing in the morning and at night to release tension.

Dynamic stretching is more of a flow, and it improves the range of our limbs' movements and increases body temperature and the speed of nerve impulses. It also accelerates our energy production and prepares our bodies for athletic activity. Stretching excites the body and prepares it for physical performance and flow. The stretch invigorates the flow of energy and prepares us for vigorous exercise. We decrease the risk of injury with dynamic stretching, as proven by both recreational and elite athletes (think of a more active or Vinyasa flow yoga).

Static and dynamic stretching

Static stretching plus dynamic stretching is the best combination of stretches for achieving optimal results for your muscles. When you combine short static stretching for no longer than six seconds with more extended dynamic stretching movements, it positively affects the muscles.

I like to combine them with my morning walk by starting with short static stretches and then opening up to more dynamic stretches mid-walk. Suppose your activity mainly involves erratic contractions, like downhill running in the mountains with the quadriceps taking the entire load. In that case, it may be helpful to dedicate some extra exercises to static stretching for those muscle sectors to stretch them out more.

Walking

Taking a nice walk at a steady pace every day benefits our hearts, joints, and posture. I have experienced the benefits firsthand and believe in the power of an excellent walk to increasingly strengthen my body and cultivate a stronger stomach and leaner waist. Then there's the benefit that these movements can provide for our minds.

Walking helps us to produce serotonin and endorphins. Serotonin is called the good mood hormone and acts as an antidepressant as well. In addition to making us happy, serotonin is a derivative of tryptophan, an amino acid that can raise melatonin production. Melatonin is a hormone produced by the pineal gland at the base of our brains, which acts on the hypothalamus glands to regulate the sleep-wake cycle.

When we move, we reduce our bodies' allopathic loads (the wear and tear on our bodies) that accumulate when exposed to repeated chronic stress. So, be mindful, get up, and walk around every twenty minutes to get your body moving. Our bodies react to being sedentary by producing cortisol, better known as the stress hormone. If we want to reduce stress, we need to move our muscles and change our thoughts.

You should try it—get up and move around right now.

Get up and move your body, even take a walk!

Research conducted by the English University of Exeter shows that a daily walk for twenty minutes can calm the nervous system, reduce hunger, and even eliminate the urge for sugar.[6] The impact is that we can develop better appetite control if we just get up and walk around.

Getting our bodies to move also spurs the creative process by stimulating the brain's frontal lobe, an area connected to creativity. After a walk or some activity, we are more mentally productive. We've got to move, walk, and stimulate our bodies to get our minds engaged, and there are physiological and psychological advantages too:

- When we exercise, our hearts pump faster, and more blood and oxygen reach our brains. That allows our brains to perform better, particularly regarding memory and attention.

- When we exercise, significant changes occur in our minds. When we find ourselves walking without requiring particular concentration, we allow our imagination to wander, and new ideas or points of view can develop.

For a healthy walk, keep up a brisk pace for at least thirty minutes without straining yourself. You can allow your heart to be active without being tired. Take advantage of a beautiful sunny day to spend some time outside to rejuvenate your body and mind. You can't stay indoors all the time, so find a place to renew your connection with the outdoors.

---

6   https://www.ncbi.nlm.nih.gov/pmc/articles/PMC7290253/

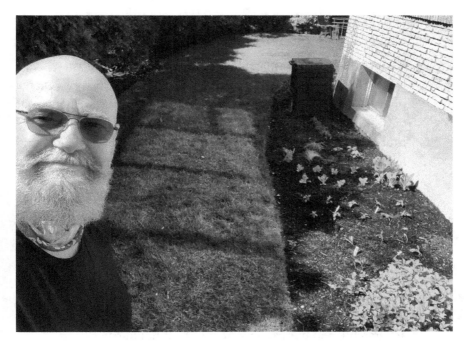

My little spice garden, Port Washington, NY

Gardening

I love working in the garden and growing healthy food, spices, and vegetables to use in our meals. You can bring a mindset of physical well-being to many activities. If you can't go anywhere, gardening is a great alternative. Gardening is one activity that is suitable if you dislike going to the gym but want to keep your body in motion. You can do it indoors or outdoors.

If you are fortunate enough to have a corner of land or even a tiny terrace large enough to hold a few pots, you can reap the benefits of caring for plants, flowers, and trees. It's a fun activity that offers exercise at any age or stage of development where movement or the range of motion might be limited.

Besides the movement, one of the desirable benefits is growing small quantities of fruits and vegetables. Many people garden primarily to make sure they are consuming quality food.

I love gardening because it is one of those activities that, besides providing genuine and straightforward satisfaction, gives me a way to exercise my muscles, joints, and mind. Here are six tangible benefits of garden care that soothe the body, mind, and spirit while connecting us to the earth, air, sunlight, and abundant nutrients that sustain and provide life.

1. **Reduces stress:** Scientific studies show that gardening is an excellent activity for reducing cortisol levels. Reducing cortisol benefits psychological well-being and also contributes to the well-being of our cardiovascular system.

2. **Motivates moderate-intensity physical activity:** Gardening involves kneeling, pulling on your arms and hands, moving medium distances, bending your back, and keeping your balance in unusual positions. Any person who hates physical activity may not willingly perform all these movements. Yet gardening offers the right incentives—seeing your garden flourish and become more beautiful can provide the proper leverage to get you into action.

3. **Training for strength and hand agility:** Anyone who has ever pruned a plant or tree knows how much power is needed to handle pruning shears. With ongoing use over time, our hands and joints are grateful, and our gardens are too. You should try it.

4. **Keeps the brain healthy:** A fascinating study from the Institutional Review Board on Cardiovascular Health Study (CHS) recruited close to a thousand participants, aged sixty-five and older. They identified gardening (practiced regularly) as one of the most efficient activities for reducing the risk of the onset of senile dementia.[7]

5. **Strengthens the immune system:** Life in the open air has benefits, and gardening is an excellent incentive to get out of the house. Exposure to direct sunlight helps our bodies get vitamin D with all its associated positive effects.

6. **Reduces the risk of depression and treats mental health:** Gardening is a beneficial activity and interest. It helps keep our minds in training to find solutions, learn new things, and share our passion with other people—all factors that contribute to our mental health. Spending a few hours in contact with nature is an excellent way to take advantage of the green grass, earth, and the spirit's healing powers.

---

7   https://pubmed.ncbi.nlm.nih.gov/8275211/

All of these benefits have been especially fruitful, especially during the pandemic. It's nice to have other interests and stay active. We must do our best to connect with nature and nurture our emotions with logic, reason, and fresh air, and we must relate to the earth, sky, water, and the elements that help nourish us.

Dancing

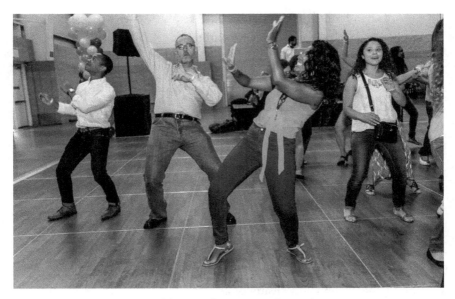

Celebrating dance at PWC, 2014

I love to dance. Dancing is a force of nature, sending its sound vibrations to electrify us with energy and vitality. Dancing has a physical and mental impact on the brain and body, impacting everyone with some movement, be it hands, feet, or sometimes other crazy manifestations.

Whether young or old, it fills dancers with vitality. There are many types of music and dance: classical, modern, funky, hip hop, Latin American, etc. What differentiates a dance from other sports is the mental component. When we dance, we allow our bodies to think and our minds to feel.

Often, we don't like getting up from the couch to go running or go to the gym or go for a swim because of the physical effort with no emotional involvement. Dance is different; some music types can influence us mentally and emotionally, stimulating us to move differently. We can do it in the living room, shower, bedroom, or anywhere—even an elevator. Listening, moving, and grooving our bodies to the beat is required.

Benefits of dancing for the body:

- It is suitable for the heart because it improves circulation, lowers blood pressure and cholesterol levels, and prevents heart attacks.

- It is handy for the muscles because aerobic activity oxygenates the blood and improves elasticity and tone.

- It trains our breath because it is anaerobic activity.

- It is an ally against stress and stimulates endorphin production and, therefore, produces pleasant sensations.

- It improves posture and is an excellent remedy for back pain.

- It stimulates the mind and memory and keeps the reflexes active.

- In older people, like me, dancing is beneficial because it can prevent Alzheimer's by keeping the mind active. It obliges us to remember steps and sequences and combats loneliness, which, unfortunately, more and more of us experience.

Dancing is also suitable for children because it helps them socialize, teaches a sense of rhythm, stimulates creativity and coordination, and keeps away the probability of developing childhood obesity.

Choosing your dance moves

With dance, the important thing is to always start with small steps. Find a partner or teacher, and you'll improve and increase your moves and intensity with time. Every age group, or generation, has its type of dance. But in reality, it's your style and physical state that dictate your moves. Whatever your age, you can try it all (ballroom dances, waltzes, tango, etc.). Dance with children and then evolve into different dance styles depending on your taste (funky, classic, modern, hip hop, etc.).

Lovers of Latin culture focus more on Latin American dances, such as salsa, bachata, merengue, samba, cha-cha, or the rumba. Then there is freestyle, to just get your "dance on," groove and move. That's the dance I practice at home when I am just listening to music or at a party with friends. There are no steps or rules for to follow, just have a fun time, swing, shake, and be well.

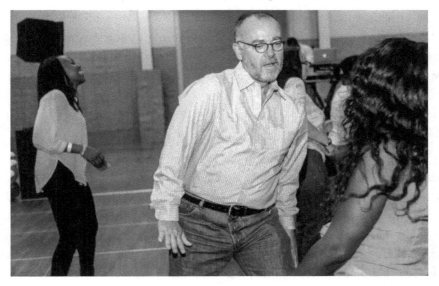

Celebrating dance at PWC Party 2014

I danced to John Travolta songs in my youth. But then Gabrielle Roth and her 5Rhythms of movement and dance emerged to remove stress and help people reconnect with life. Gabrielle Roth created the 5Rhythms dance course in the 1970s. I think of her to be the founding mother of all Conscious Dance practices. The 5Rhythms are like an emotional road map, a template or mandala, to explore movement—move in, out, forward, back, in the physical, emotional, and intellectual realms. 5Rhythms music connects us to the wisdom of our bodies, freeing us and moving us into a dynamic and healing movement as meditation, energetic medicine, and ecstatic devotional prayer. Moving our bodies helps us feel balanced and connected. With Conscious Dance practices, we get to emote, move, and shake to life's rhythms.

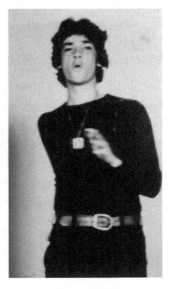

Acting school, Lee Strasberg, 1972

Dancing the 5Rhythms uses music that evokes emotional states as a tool to rediscover our primal ancestral heritage through movement.

The 5Rhythms are flowing, staccato, chaos, lyrical, and stillness. Together they correspond to the five steps that return us to our inner balance and help us understand the energy we may experience at a specific time. Flowing and staccato favor the connection with feminine and masculine energy. Chaos corresponds to the maximum expression of our vital lives, while lyrical stimulates a state of trance in which it is possible to penetrate the mysteries of being. Finally, with stillness, we return home to our inner lives.

There are no specific steps to learn for 5Rhythms. It is a method of free body expression structured with five phases and five types of rhythmic music. Their rhythms range from slow and Tai-Chi-like to wild and chaotic. We speak of "dancing waves" in the 5Rhythms. A *flowing* rhythm is a soft and circular motion that can then turn into *staccato's* sharp and well-defined moves. Then there is the *chaos* movement, where one can shake or dance wildly. The *lyrical* dance is light and cheerful, which can then slow down to the delicate movements of *stillness*. Then we stop, and the cycle of the 5Rhythms is finished. After one wave, we could start another one right away. Dancing a wave is liberating, balancing, and calming.

Effects and benefits of the 5Rhythms

The dance of the 5Rhythms is adaptable for all ages and situations. It combines the benefits of movement with meditation and awakening the body, mind, and spirit. On a physical level, it increases flexibility, strengthens the muscles, and stimulates circulation. It also helps to rest the mind and reduce stress and anxiety. Each rhythm is interpreted by individuals in unique and personal ways, opening them up to a new sense of freedom and possibility that is surprising, healing, exhilarating, and profoundly regenerating. It is an exercise for the right brain.

Lifting Weights

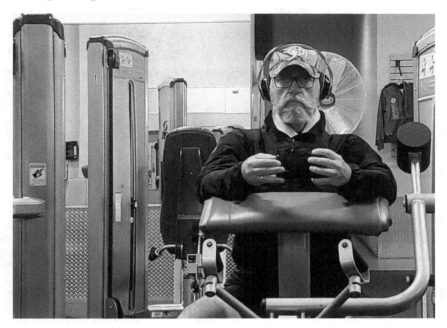

Taking weight training too seriously. Training Station, Port Washington, NY 2017

Building muscle is important, especially as we get older. Cardiovascular health includes lifting weights, stretching, and aerobic exercises for maximum benefit. It takes effort to lift weights, and it benefits the heart, so it's an important endeavor to undertake, slowly and gradually.

The primary goal of weight training is to define and strengthen the muscles. Posture and form are essential to a healthy walk, body frame, and gait. It is vital, like anything else, to start slowly and increase the weights gradually for maximum performance.

When we combine weights with aerobic exercise, before or after an aerobic routine (on a treadmill or an exercise bike, for example), we get the combined benefits of helping our muscles and heart. As we develop the routine, we build endurance. Resting, burning fat, and building resistance sum up the training we want to put in place. By creating a routine with weights, we reduce the risk associated with osteoporosis. Weights improve posture, increase strength, and help us avoid losing muscle mass. These are essential requirements as we age due to a loss of bone density. We need muscle to stand taller, continue to be in tip-top shape, and have the necessary energy flowing into our bodies as we age.

Many people avoid weight training for fear of getting hurt or disproportionately increasing their muscles. If we don't want muscle mass, we focus on tone. Our perspective dictates the approach we take. If we learn the proper techniques, we can change our view by adjusting the workout. We can lift weights according to our abilities and goals.

Lifting weights has many benefits. Besides those already mentioned, it improves health, allows us to age better, helps prevent injuries, increases blood flow, and helps us enjoy a better quality of life.

To get all of the advantages, go beyond lifting dumbbells and incorporate movement during your session to vary it. A high-intensity weightlifting routine with a series of ten movement repetitions for each can increase your body's oxygen levels and improve circulation.

Seven tips to help start your weightlifting routine

1. Take five to ten minutes to warm up and cool down before and after your workout. Take a walk or use the stretching exercises mentioned earlier.
2. Take the time to align, define, and refine your body to the moves. Visualize the movement and go slowly for the repetitions. Manage your breath and concentrate on slow, smooth lifts and equally controlled descents while isolating a muscle group.
3. Create the right tempo and breathe into the movement to stay in control rather than compromise strength gains with momentum. For example, count to three while lowering a weight, hold, and then count to three while raising it to the starting position.
4. Pay attention to your breath. Exhale as you work against the resistance by lifting, pushing, or pulling; inhale as you release.
5. Slowly increase the weight or resistance. When you add weight, remember to do all the repetitions with the proper form, and the targeted muscles should feel tired by the last two.
6. Create a routine. Working all the body's major muscles two or three times a week is ideal.

7. Take time off to let your muscles heal, repair, and grow stronger. Take at least forty-eight hours to recover before your next strength-training session.

Staying Fit

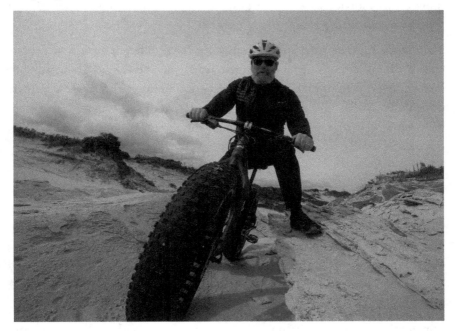

South Africa Dirt Bike, 2018

Staying fit is the primary goal of body mindfulness. It helps us balance and get back to the essential nature of our mind, body, and spirit connections.

If you don't fancy going to the gym, whatever the reason, there are alternatives. First, decide that you are going to get in shape. Don't compare and despair because you are old, skinny, fat, or don't like the smell of sweat, workout music, or the general sound of exercise. Don't let the gym or the lack of an exercise room ruin your true intentions.

You can take charge of your physical life with a mindful intention that says, "I will pay attention to my body." By keeping your focus on the benefits of physical activity, you can reinforce the purpose with a declaration saying, "I want to live strong and long for many years to come." By staying fit, you gain vigor and the ability to be independent in your later years. But how do you keep fit without going to the gym?

Believe it or not, it is mind over matter

A study by Erin M. Shackell and Lionel G. Standing at Bishop's University showed that individuals who didn't exercise could create gains in strength and fitness without lifting a finger!

Their study measured the strength gains for three different groups of people. Group One did nothing outside their usual routine. Group Two was put through two weeks of highly focused strength training for one specific muscle three times a week. Group Three just listened to audio CDs that guided them to imagine that they were going through the same workout as Group Two, three times a week.

Visualization

Group One, which did nothing, saw no gains in strength. The exercise group, Group Two, trained three times a week and saw a 28 percent gain in strength. The visualization group, Group Three, visualized exercising, and they experienced improvements in their physical power and strength by 24 percent. They received almost the same benefit in terms of strength gains as the group that worked out!

Apparently, through visualization, our bodies respond, and we increase strength. How it works remains a mystery to me and many others. We need to incorporate visualization into our strength-training arsenal. Shackell noted that "Studies like this one reinforce the reality that our mental and physical systems are very much connected and can influence each other."[8]

Six get fit ideas

Many activities help us get fit and be well. With a minimum effort and will-power and a bit of physical exertion, we can incorporate these into our daily routines to see the benefits.

---

8   Erin M. Shackell and Lionel G. Standing, North American Journal of Psychology 9, no.1 (2007): 189–200.

1. **Ban elevators**—Don't avoid the stairs in a building or during your morning commute. Climbing stairs is an exercise that helps keep you in shape as much as a gym machine.

2. **Grocery lifting**—Whether you do it weekly or every two or three days, go shopping on foot (distances permitting) and carry your groceries.

3. **Clean**—I love this one especially. You can combine your visualization of exercise with house cleaning. Just imagine yourself exercising every part of your body while you are cleaning. Get into it, and you will have a healthier body and a cleaner home.

4. **Take a walk**—Walking at least half an hour a day is one way toward a healthy life. You can stroll or walk fast and do it for an hour or longer (perhaps using fitness-walking techniques). You can also go to the park early in the morning, before going to work, or in the evening.

5. **Walk the dog**—Walking the dog is a persuasive reason to leave home and take a walk in the countryside. Do not delegate this task, especially if it's your dog.

6. **Pedal**—Get on a bicycle and take a short trip. It's a fun activity that is not just for the young because every age can do it. It also promotes balance and hand-eye coordination.

Tech Fitness

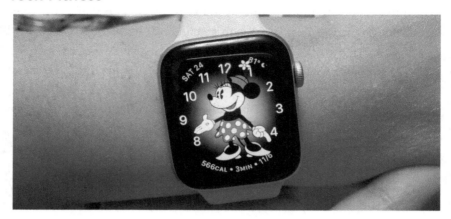

My Niece's Apple/Health Fitness Watch

Whatever you need, there is a gadget for it. Tech fitness is increasingly essential. With the iPhone, Apple Watch (with Minnie Mouse too), Samsung, and Garmin, many companies have moved into the healthcare space for remote diagnostics. The focus is to log, track, and design routines to maximize steps, food, caloric intake, and get the users motivated about life. They can now provide ongoing respiration, heartbeat, and blood sugar levels.

You can monitor your health with sensors that detect heart rate, UV rays, sweating, and more. Do you want accurate calculations on the number of calories you've burned and the related recovery times? You can even monitor your progress and know which vitamins to take to increase vitality and boost your immune system.

Smartwatches today can notify us when a sudden drop in blood pressure happens, showing that we may need to deal with a severe heart attack. With real-time monitoring of the pulse, heart rate, and blood pressure, it's like having a nursing assistant with us at all times. It's all available to use with the click of a button.

Do you want a better night's sleep? By monitoring your sleep at night, you can capture valuable data to improve sleep quality. The technology will also wake you up in the morning with confidence that you will feel refreshed.

Not everyone can have a personal trainer who will follow them seven days a week. Still, tech offers us a way to actively and mindfully manage what we eat, the exercises we do, and the ones we have to perform to reach a specific target. Devices equipped with a heart-rate monitor allow us to check how tired or toned our muscles should be and which liquids are needed to keep our bodies and minds refreshed.

> *My daily workout involves walking two miles. This is where I stop,*
> *stretch, reflect on my motivations, and give thanks for the day.*

Motivation and Objectives

So, let's recap this chapter. You've looked at the various ways to stretch your mind, body, and spirit, either at the gym, during activities, or by using visualization. How or when you stretch or do a workout is up to you.

Choose your sport with focus, commitment, and discipline. Be mindful and passionate about carrying out your daily mission focused on feeling positive and living life to its fullest. You will need to adopt an attitude of commitment to change and resolve to use discipline to meet your challenges. Create a plan that will help you move forward based on your age, physical condition, and effort. Every day, small steps will enable you to take a long journey over the weeks, months, and years ahead.

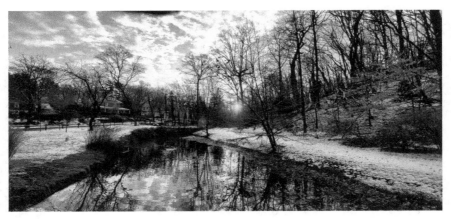

My morning walk motivation, Port Washington, NY

Whatever your motivation, you will have the best results if you visualize the results. Write your reasons. Answer the what, when, where, how, and why questions. If you choose to walk, run, lift weights, play sports, or play with your grandchildren, do it with a sense of fun, pleasure, passion, and determination. You'll get better results.

Here's some guidance to help you go forward.

- If your goal is to tone your muscles, swimming is the best choice.

- If weight loss is your goal, the most popular options are yoga, aerobic courses, walking or fit walking, cycling, and running.

- If pure fun is your motivation, and you have a proper sense of rhythm, try dance, rumba, or another program that starts in the shower and moves to your gym's dance floor.

- Choose a team sport like baseball, soccer, volleyball, rugby, or basketball if you can find a local team. You might discover wonderful friendships there too.

- Finally, if you are up to it and feel like expressing your animal side, you can try CrossFit or even pole dancing.

- Training with others will motivate you. Competition is part of our nature. But individual training allows you to manage your time. As you get older and involved with work, family, and responsibilities, you may not have the time.

Mindfulness of the body requires that you have discipline and commitment. It is necessary to be mindful. Working out by yourself requires putting yourself on a regular schedule. I start my day at 5 a.m. I meditate, replenish my liquids, and then go to the gym, or during these days of COVID-19, I go for a 2-mile walk around my neighborhood, with a stretch in the middle. How do you want to start your routine?

What days can you commit to, and when can you do it? Remember that it takes twenty-eight days to make a habit and three days to break it. So, what are you going to commit to doing? What challenges will you face? How will you handle those challenges? Plan for the challenges and be ready to give yourself compassion and a boost of loving-kindness for starting. Then get back on the treadmill of life.

Mindful Tips

Do not overdo it! You only want a workout—not burnout. Set a regular target to reach. Keep records from the first day of training. Use your watch, smartphone, or another device (paper and pencil) to note your progress, one week to the next. Gradually progress.

Do not get discouraged. Go back repeatedly, acknowledge the challenge, and do it anyway. Challenge is necessary for the training. As you may remember, it's mind over matter. Your new physical form will take shape gradually. Ensure that you consult your doctor. Undertake a gradual path to achieve your results, and respect your body and your possibilities. Visualize the results.

Finally, remember that you have signed no blood pact or bond to stay with it. If you realize an activity is not suitable for you, go back to the visualization, determine your motivation, and look for another, more satisfying one.

There are no more excuses. All you have to do is start practicing the sport or activity you've always wanted and start living a mindful, more aware relationship with your body.

How do you rate yourself?

Body: *Energy and Flexibility.*

Are you active? Do you move your muscles and include movement and physical activities, like walking, dancing, gardening, sports, lifting weights, yoga, cycling, swimming, and working out in a gym, into your daily, weekly routines?

How do you rate yourself on a scale of 1 (low) to 5 (high)?

Where are you?

1	2	3	4	5

Where do you want to be?

1	2	3	4	5

Why did you choose this number?

_____

_____

_____

What changes could you make to help you get there?

_____

_____

_____

Source: Personal Health Inventory –

Veterans Affairs. https://www.va.gov/WHOLEHEALTH/docs/10-773_PHI_May2020.pdf

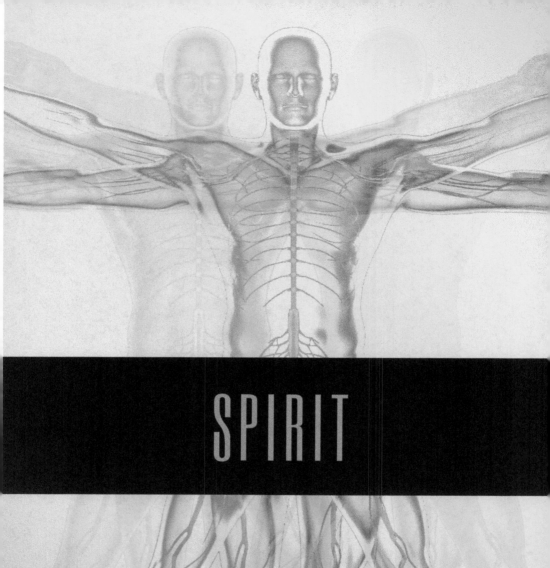

SPIRIT

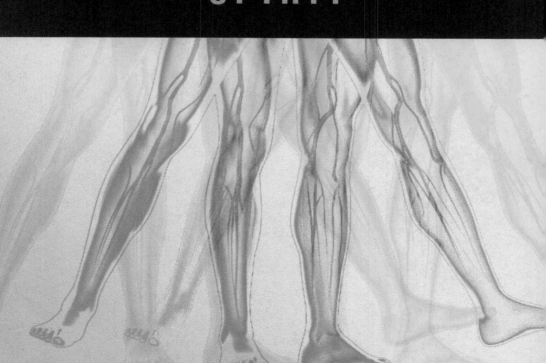

Chapter 3

SPIRIT

Growing and Connecting

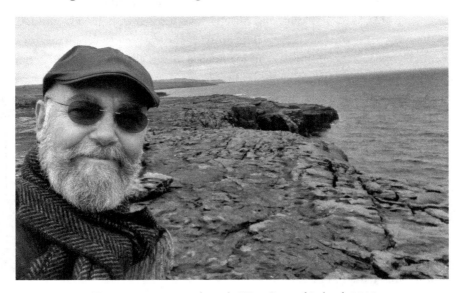

Tracing my ancestry, along the West Coast of Ireland, 2019

BE STILL AND know that I AM. Ask yourself, "Why was I born?" or "Why am I here?" or "What is the purpose of my life?" Investigation of these questions is the focus of this chapter.

Questions like these evoke a sense of concern, interest, or fear for many of us. They call upon us to wake up, find meaning, purpose, appreciation, and even compassion for what I call "sacred moments of truth."

When things are hard, where do we turn to for strength and comfort? Spiritual or religious faith, prayers, meditation, nature, art, music? Or do you prefer quiet time alone, on a walk perhaps? Some want to help others, to connect with meaningful experiences while serving those in need. How do we express our sense of a higher power to find meaning and purpose in our lives? There are spirit and soul guides outside of our culture's materialism that nourish us and help us look at life so we can fully live it. You can find these spirit guides in the wind, the sky, the earth under your feet, or in a bird's cry. You can find them in the waves that crash along the shore or the koi swimming in a calm pond. You can find them in the fire's roar on a snowy day or the sound of the kettle awaiting you with a cup of hot tea.

We all try to understand our lives by looking for a sense of meaning and purpose in them. We tell our own stories, histories, and mythologies. We have heroes, villains, warriors, kings and queens, lovers, sorrows, betrayals, and reconciliations. Our time on this earth is limited, and we seek to create meaning through concepts, perspectives, and ideological views, all of which impact our perceptions and waking moments. Our thoughts provide us with pathways forward, offering us hope, intrigue, and even terror. Our views affect how we deal with the world and how we help ourselves and others.

Who are we? Culturally, we fashion ourselves based on archetypes and social narratives, the mythologies, stars, and heroes that resonate with us. These are the historical mythologies, legends, and heroes who fought battles against all odds, who won in sports, music, politics, business and religion. We value these stories and myths about what is essential, in ourselves and society (the successful wife, husband, business entrepreneur, etc.) and compare and measure our worth accordingly. Using those narratives as templates, we form a story about who we are or wish to be.

But what if these narratives, the stories and things we relied upon, no longer work? What if we find ourselves empty of energy in an unknown place, and the familiar stories or images don't work for us? How do we find meaning, then? By turning inward, toward a spiritual or religious path, or finding comfort in nature among the rivers, streams, mountains, valleys, oceans, and trees, many find solace and relief from the world's burdens.

When things fall apart, as they will, how do you connect with your inner spirit, your soul?
Service is the highest form of worship

—Debasish Mridha

Some find their connections to a higher calling by helping others in service to a deeper calling in life. They find humility, insights, and links to spirit guides that present profound and more in-depth questions about life and death. We are touched, moved, and inspired to realize that what flows through others flows through us. We find our mission and calling to be of service and interconnected in a cosmic dance of space and time. We come to know that when we are of service to others, we replenish and renew our energies and connections with all of life.

Being connected with ourselves and others helps us ignite our spirits' and souls' yearnings and unlock our deepest aspirations. First, we find depth and meaning as we cultivate our minds and bodies. We develop a close, personal relationship with our breath, our thoughts, our feelings, sensations, and the feeling of the blood flowing through our bodies as we exercise and stretch. (Please refer to chapter 2 for specific stretches and exercises.)

By being grounded, we are better able to access our mission on Earth. We open ourselves to receiving directions from our inner GPS, which guides us toward our soul's yearnings, our life's mission, a higher purpose—asking ourselves questions requires input to determine who, what, when, how, and why we are here. We become activists, cultivating this personal relationship with ourselves and then with people, places, and things. All of these help us think, learn, and grow.

Having this ongoing relationship with ourselves, our breath, and the world is the essence of mindfulness. When we can anchor ourselves to our breath, we can see the world more clearly, moment by moment, and cut through the noise and chatter to hear our thoughts more clearly. We gain the wisdom needed to act with kindness and compassion and venture into the world to explore it and learn from it as we engage with the environment we encounter. We can alter our old worn-out belief systems because we accept our stories and the people who did whatever they did and be at peace about them. We can then evolve, transform, and strip away the dust and debris from the old narratives that cover the spirit's true nature.

The Essence of Spirituality

I believe that the difference between religion and spirituality is like the difference between the menu and the meal. Religion is the menu; spirituality is the meal. On the religion menu, there are various ethnic choices, different spices, flavors, and ingredients. Spirituality is the meal, served like the breath and the wind. Its essence is not tangible, but its meaning and power have influenced the spoken word and the course of lives over the centuries. Many religious people are also spiritual, but many are not. They follow the precepts without connecting them to their nature, humanity, and sensing no interconnectedness with people who do not believe what they do.

Our spirituality provides us with consciousness, presence, and the spirit to get up and be in the world. It gives us the aspiration and inspiration to make the world a better place for ourselves and others.

Spiritually active people know how to think, love, and work. If you are a person without a spiritual life, you may feel powerless and exposed to every danger, like an animal deprived of its instinct. Having a spiritual life is like having a command center for human life. Hormones may regulate the body, and awareness may give dimension to the psyche, but having a conscience might provide moral sensitivity. However, all spheres of personal existence come into view with a spiritual life and our interconnectedness to other human beings, regardless of their religious beliefs.

Spirituality offers us a broader path, whether it's Judaism, Christianity, Buddhism, Taoism, Islam, Atheism, or Animism. Whatever our sacred way might be, its myths and stories can be very different and yet the same—stories of faith, hope, love, and despair tell us that the spirit goes forward. It battles to know death and rebirth and to better understand our interconnectedness with good, evil, trial, tribulation, and redemption.

Religion without spirituality

Fundamentalists have religious beliefs that stop them from appreciating the religious beliefs of others. It is strange and hard for them to respect others who do not think the same as they do or grasp the same ideals, myths, or stories. Fundamentalists have a strong sense of the importance of maintaining the distinction between themselves and others; their inherent bias rejects the application of opinion and diversity to specific "fundamentals" and their accepted interpretation of an unbendable set of beliefs. Not seeing any interconnectedness between themselves and others, they often put themselves beyond the reach of others, emotionally, spiritually, and intellectually. Their views isolate them, leaving them afraid and often angry. They feel they must fight the growing tide of progressive change that interprets religious beliefs and God through the lenses of an increasing population inhabiting the earth.

Neglected Spirituality

Increasingly, we live in a global society that values materialism, the acquisition of wealth, goods, and services more than the accumulation of virtue, merit, and good deeds. So, are people with a lot of money and "stuff" happier? The answer may surprise you. Researchers have found that more money does not yield much more happiness at all above a certain point. A Harvard study of the money-happiness relationship[9] shows that money matters for well-being, but there is no difference in satisfaction between people with family incomes of $50,000 and $75,000. Once your basic needs are fulfilled (food, shelter, and clothing), happiness is an inside job that builds upon your relationship with yourself and the relationships you have with people, places, and things. There are many reasons why people without money are happier than those with lots of it. Those without money have an expanded sense of gratitude and humility than those with lots of it.

It is more likely that a child will ask their parents for something to eat rather than something to meditate upon or a "pearl of wisdom" to nourish their spirit's yearning for growth. While recent trends have looked at the role of yoga, and its industry has grown as a path to exercise and mindfulness, it

---

9   https://www.pnas.org/content/107/38/16489.full

focuses on boosting physical tone and mental productivity. Spirituality is not prominent in most Western cultures. Many people (young, middle-aged, and older) don't ask themselves the eternal questions, for example, "Why am I here?" They live unexamined lives.

What do we need? Food, shelter, clothing, sleep, and hopefully someone who loves us, who we can care for and love. Yet, in our race to the top, we often put aside personal relationships, sacrificing them to work so we can earn more and get more "stuff." We don't have the time for those who genuinely lift us. Have you heard the saying, "Some people know the price of everything and the value of nothing?" It's very appropriate for many people stuck in consumer culture. Many get so caught up with their net worth—which they perceive dictates their self-worth—that they don't have time for others. Comparing and despairing over a particular car, house, or fashion item is crazy. We cannot find happiness by grasping and groping in the pursuit of wealth.

Quantum physics and the law of attraction theorists claim we are all connected from our internal energy fields to the outside world. Like batteries, we are all connected through an energy field that permeates the ether. Beyond our physical bodies is an energy universe connecting us all in a subtle web and interconnecting us in time and space. Throughout Indian, Taoist, and Tibetan cultures, there is the concept that our formlessness and subtle bodies are wired into this energy field of existence. We can call this subtle body a spirit body.

Studies of Chinese medicine, acupuncture specifically, focus on the body's meridians and acupoints, points that can be open to or block energy. Acupuncture helps open these points and can suppress pain during significant surgery. Our gross physical bodies know how to interpret physical impulses and need to survive, eat, stay warm, and be happy. In Buddhist tantra, this subtle body is called our "innate body," and it comprises thousands of subtle energy channels (*nadis*). These energy channels are conduits for energies or "winds" (lung or prana).

The three main nadis—central, left, and right—run from the point between the eyebrows up to the crown chakra and down through all seven chakras to end two inches below the navel. These areas of the body give rise to energy, which gives rise to form. We human beings are more than skin bags made of

60 percent water and chemicals. But if we think of ourselves only as a physical body that consumes, eats, wakes, sleeps, and propagates the species, we ignore our true nature. We cannot transcend the physical plane of reality if we live with a survival mentality.

Transcendence requires that it fully embodies us, that we let go of what we've become, to reemerge into a state of emptiness. Transcendence requires that we trust the process, that we have faith in the higher frequencies of love and compassion, rather than being slaves to lower base impulses (fear and doubt). It means that we develop our abilities to become masters of our experience and wise guides to our inner and outer spheres of influence. By cultivating a spiritual life, being present to our breath and each moment-by-moment experience, we can develop this higher frequency. We can visualize our changing world. With positive intentions for ourselves and all living beings, we can put these intentions into the world, to create our reality, with our body, speech, and minds. All this starts when we ask ourselves what life means and how we can shape our lives and the world in the present moment.

As human beings, we are both form and formless. We are always becoming. Like verbs and nouns, we act with intention and see the potentialities projected and formed into the world. The work of Albert Einstein, Louis de Broglie, and many others established that all objects have both wave and particle nature (though this is only detectable on a minute scale, such as with atoms). Quantum mechanics provides the overarching theory resolving this apparent paradox. Each breath we breathe, each thought and action we take, can transport us into the intended present moments of our becoming.

Our essential nature is both form and formless, particle and wave. We are pure potential, only bound by time and space. We have only so many breaths to breathe our potential, to visualize and be present with what is possible in our lives, right here and right now. We have to ask, "How can I bring my gifts into the world to benefit myself and others?" We then need to have faith that we can materialize our gifts through our actions.

Spiritual Bypassing

In the early 1980s, John Welwood, a Buddhist teacher and psychotherapist, introduced the term *spiritual bypassing* to describe how many people use spiritual ideas and practices to sidestep unresolved emotional issues, psychological wounds, and unfinished developmental tasks.

I've seen this in my development over the years and in others. Those deep issues, traumas, and problems hurt too much, and somehow, we believe if we don't look at an issue, it will go away. We believe that religion or spirituality will "wash clean" the sins of the past and clean the wreckage of our lives. We also think that it will help us feel better emotionally and spiritually "save us" from the emotional or psychic pain of what happened. We might act as if nothing happened or that we are over it and invest in decorating our homes, buying statues, going to church or a temple, or even hugging a tree out into nature. But we need to do the work and come to grips with our narrative around those incidents, to understand, accept, and embrace our stories. Mindfulness exercises might help, and we might indeed experience the traumatic incidents again as we practice concentrating. Mindfulness practices offer us valuable ways to support our connections and aspire toward a higher plane of existence.

Spiritual Maturity

A spiritually mature person can reflect, love, and understand that they cannot be the center of the universe, or go it alone. They know they need others, and they plug into a web of interconnected, energetic beings to find health, wellness, and happiness. By connecting they can reflect their insides to others on the outside. We see them for the people they are on the inside, and we share an energetic vibrational hug. Like the air we breathe, spirit hides in plain sight, yet it empowers our inspirations, aspirations, or finds us desperate and expired when we don't connect to it.

The word *sonder* is defined as "the realization that each random passerby is living a life as vivid and complex as our own, populated with their ambitions, friends, routines, worries, and inherited craziness."10 It is an insightful concept and helps us live spiritual lives. An epic story continues invisibly around us. It's like being in an anthill sprawling deep underground, with elaborate passageways to thousands of other lives that we never knew existed. This is what being connected means. Much of humanity lives with the illusion of separateness. The only way to overcome this illusion and its resultant loneliness is to remember our connectedness and commit to living with empathy and compassion. What I do to another is invariably done to me.

When we explore our higher natures, our cosmic selves, and the aspirational self that arises from our hopes, dreams, and wishes, we ask questions and seek answers. We discover that serenity is within our reach and that we can trust in ourselves and the surrounding supporting universe. We can bring together an awareness of our bodies, minds, memories, impulses, instincts, and emotions that define our past. When we find acceptance, it gifts us with the present moment and the possibility of finding real potential in a continually unfolding future. When we consider those who have helped us along the way, like our mothers who have cared for us with love, kindness, or friendship, we can further recognize our blessings and be present for ourselves and others.

10   https://www.dictionaryofobscuresorrows.com/post/23536922667/sonder

Mother to All Beings

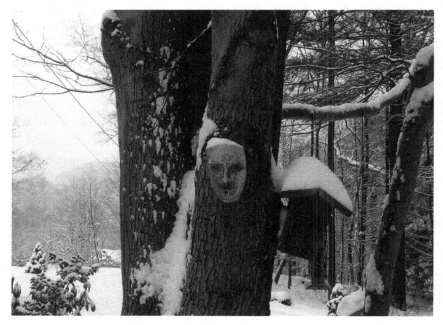

Mother earth, our favorite tree, Pond Eddy, NY, 2010

As a father and grandfather, I can tell you that being a parent requires the most extraordinary spiritual sacrifices. Parents give and receive love to raise a child. They work, sweat, and toil for another human being; I can give no more tremendous sacrifice or gift. A spiritually mature person knows that without love, life becomes an incomprehensible, unbearable void. With a commitment to life and the love that comes from it, we can devote ourselves to benefit others in this world by being a Mother to All Beings.

We can adopt a motherly attitude of love and gratitude and see all living beings deserving of love like ourselves—including wildlife, green plants, fish in the sea, and even insects. When we live and grow spiritually, we are open to encountering higher powers, energetic forces of nature, like the breath that breathes in all sapient beings. It is the breath, the spirit, that offers us hope and faith in times of darkness and despair, pain, and misery. Be it in the deep waters of South Africa or the rich green forests of Brazil, we find strength in everything alive.

What does it mean to find your strength? We find our strength in our abilities to overcome, survive, and lean into our weak moments with compassion that nourishes and cares for us. Thinking, feeling, and visualizing are the skills that distinguish us as human beings. We can face tough times and navigate through the rough waters of life, the terrible storms and situations that throw us off course, and then find our place in the world.

Think about it. Our ancestors survived and thrived. We were born into this world with the power to succeed. In our DNA and bloodstreams, we have the chemistry to endure and overcome all the challenges that life might put before us. Knowing this, we can have faith that we will find the courage to move forward during disastrous times, even though we cannot see ahead. With that faith, we can conceive success, believe in it, then realize and actualize it with motivation. Even when life falters and everything becomes dark, we can shine a light, an image, into the darkness, and with faith, we can find our way despite the pain or obstacles that afflict us. We can find resilience. Our capacities to endure have no limits, as long as we are breathing.

We are not alone

Many of us live in crowded cities but find ourselves alone. Many find themselves in intimate relationships but feel alone. Why? Is it because we allow ourselves to be intimate, open, imperfect, hurt, mad, sad, or scared? Vulnerability can be very frightening. Family, social, and work systems break down, become corrupt, create havoc and pain, and are indifferent. But remember, we are all interconnected; we are interdependent. We must trust each other for kindness, help, goods, and services.

Many people are in pain and numb it through drinking, drugging, eating, sex, spending, swiping, and screening. We are all coping with emotional, psychological, and physical pain, including those right next to us in the supermarket line. We gain strength from knowing that we are not alone; the human condition is that we are all dealing with some kind of suffering. Finding the courage to ask for help, allowing ourselves to be guided, and trusting with compassion require strength and determination.

When we allow others to help us be in fellowship, to share our fears and uncertainties, we allow ourselves to hold the hand of a person who might have gone down the same road as us. We have faith that our fears and uncertainties will pass. We must never stop believing because small things can happen, day by day, to change the course of our lives and bring us closer to personal satisfaction and clarity.

Things to take to heart:

- Continue to strive and find the resources within our bodies, minds, and spirits, to hear, see, and believe in our potential.

- Believe that everything will balance itself. There is no end without a beginning, no light without darkness; everything moves in cycles. Challenges make us grow. When we find the balance point and are resilient, we will come back stronger.

We need to get up, blow the dust off, and keep walking because it's worth it. Remember that life continues, time passes, and we will be the ones to tell our stories the way we want to tell them.

Don't Quit

When things go wrong, as they sometimes will,
When the road you're trudging seems all uphill,
When the funds are low and the debts are high
And you want to smile, but you have to sigh,
When care is pressing you down a bit,
Rest if you must, but don't you quit.
Life is strange with its twists and turns
As every one of us sometimes learns
And many a failure comes about
When he might have won had he stuck it out;
Don't give up though the pace seems slow—
You may succeed with another blow.
Success is failure turned inside out—
The silver tint of the clouds of doubt,
And you never can tell just how close you are,
It may be near when it seems so far;
So stick to the fight when you're hardest hit—
It's when things seem worst that you must not quit.

JOHN GREENLEAF WHITTIER.
This poem is in the public domain

Balancing Negativity—Eleven Key Ideas

Sooner or later, we all experience feelings of defeat and failure, and we cannot find meaning in our lives. These eleven key ideas focus on balancing the negative feelings, accentuating them with the positive side of life.

1. Focus on the positive side of life

Undoubtedly, there are many positive things in our lives, but just at this moment, perhaps we are blinded by negativity. Could things be different? An excellent way to discover what is positive is to make a list. When we are feeling sick and tired of life, we can take out our list and read it. Life is not what it is but how we feel it is.

2. Change your story to change your life

When something terrible is happening, we need to remember that we are still the writers of our own stories. No one else can tell us who we are unless we let them. Nothing lasts forever, not happiness, sadness, or misfortune. Our personal story has multiple, colored nuances and chapters. It could be the story of a victor who overcomes hardship, not the story of a victim… you get to choose.

3. Tomorrow is another day

In difficult moments, remember that "Tomorrow is another day" or you can always sing that famous line: "Tomorrow, tomorrow, I love you, tomorrow; you're only a day away." We can say, "Tomorrow will be a great relief, I have faith, hope, and courage to make the changes needed."

4. Recognize, rectify, and make amends

If we have made a mistake at work with a partner or friend, we can apologize and hug them instead of mulling over the issue. It is simple, and we solve the problem.

5. Surround yourself with positive people

Those surrounded by positive people see everything differently. They can talk about their problems, laugh about them, and solve them.

6. Look for solutions within yourself, not outside yourself

You are the only one who has the power to change your mind and directly change your point of view as a result. Change your story, and you can change your life.

7. You are not unusual

You are not the only one to suffer negative things or experiences. Recognize this, and you will feel less dramatic about yourself or your problems. Realize you are not alone and know that others can share your challenges.

8. Do something you like doing

Move a muscle and change a thought. When faced with challenges, don't just sit on the sofa and think about your problems. Channel your energies into your body and put your body into motion. Go out and get some fresh air and sun.

9. Get physical

Get out of your head and into your body. Go outdoors and do some physical activity, dance, or walk. Doing that at least three times a week is an excellent outlet. Follow your own pace, but you should attempt to include some activity in your life that is physical.

10. Flip the script

Flip the script of "I can't" or "I'm unlucky" to positive phrases, like "Tomorrow will be better" or "How happy and satisfied I will feel when I can overcome everything thanks to my inner strength" or "What happened will help me mature. Everything happens for a reason." Flip the script and be your own best cheerleader!

11. Believe in yourself

Be tenacious, and trust that your actions will help you. Things often change. Don't be discouraged. Look at life as a challenge that you can learn from and enjoy every moment. One day you will have bragging rights to talk about the challenges you've overcome. Life is difficult. But having inner strength and learning to manage your emotional intelligence can be a superb help.

With these eleven tips, we can infuse ourselves with the power and courage needed to overcome anything because "when we close one door, another one opens." There is always an opposite side to which we can look to for inspiration.

From the Microcosm to the Macrocosm

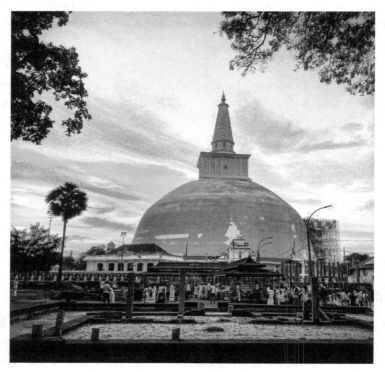

On Pilgrimage, Thuparama Seya, Sri Lanka 2019

"From the microcosm to the macrocosm" represents the balance of the universe. Its energetic influences are like those of "As above, so below." But what does that mean, and how do we apply it to our own lives?

There are over seven billion people on the planet; we each have our reality or way of seeing the world. The term *microcosm* (from the Greek *mikros kosmos* or "little world") is a Western philosophical term designating that humans are a "little world" unto themselves in which the macrocosm, or universe, is reflected. Plato's ancient Greek idea of a world soul animating the universe had a corollary—the idea that each human body is a miniature universe animated by its own soul. This concept is supported by quantum theory, which shows that we humans each create our own universe and reality, given the causes, conditions, and internal processes we undergo. We must accept responsibility for our views of the world, along with the responsibility for changing our world based on those views.

I do not limit the power of perception and projection to our own realities, causes, or conditions within the microcosm of our existence. These views have a direct impact on the reality of our existence, the macrocosm. If we change our vision of life and take responsibility for our actions and thoughts, we can change the world through our perceptions and project our light onto what we hope will be in the world. We are responsible for everything that happens in our lives. When we understand that our actions and thoughts directly influence our lives and the lives of others, our thoughts become prodigious arbitrators of what is or is not acceptable. After that, a paradigm shift happens. When we change our beliefs, we change our lives and the lives of others.

We don't need a shamanic journey or retreat on a mountain to make this shift. Being in nature or solitude can help. However, it is more about knowing that we can shift our thinking and beliefs right here and now, given our conditions. For that, we need to be honest and accept right here and now whatever is showing up for us and be willing to be the change we wish to see.

This concept of "being right here and now" took me a while to understand before I integrated it and made it mine. Only the present moment exists. It is not the past and not the future. We can use it to project into the past and build a narrative around it. Or we can project it into the future and look at what is possible. We often use a "constructive memory" to create a narrative of past or future events, infused with our accumulated lenses of hopes, fears, biases, and uncertainties. Constructive memory creates inner discomforts or regrets about what we did or didn't do in the past or anxieties about what we must do. The narratives around these are constructs that can be changed. By being present to ourselves, we can adjust the stories to generate a present and future that will benefit ourselves and others with a spirit of compassion.

Living life from the inside out

Over the past twenty-seven years, while I've done both outer and inner research, I have deepened my spiritual and philosophical connection and path. It has led me to study many of the great masters of spiritual and philosophical thought, the world's religious paths, and the common messages among all religions, which have fascinated and informed me.

I studied the messages of Jesus, Buddha, the ancient Vedic texts; and many enlightened beings, like Paramhansa Yogananda, Sri Swami Satchidananda, Osho; the Saints; writers like Freud and Jung; scientists; historical figures; mystics; and philosophers like Giordano Bruno, Meister Eckhart, David Bohm, Joseph Campbell, and others. Through my studies, I created a bridge between spirituality and science and became more aware of their complementary nature. Just as certainty requires uncertainty, spirituality can rely on science.

In my journey, I was determined to discover my purpose, why I came into the world, the "dream of my soul." When I realized this was the wrong question to ask—that it was ego driven—I asked myself other questions: "What can I do for the other people?" "How can I do it better?" "What are my talents?" Once I started asking questions this way, my life moved in a different direction.

The energetic techniques that I have practiced over the years, especially yoga and meditation, have also helped me physically and intuitively. They've helped me open perceptions previously unseen by my mind's eye—the idea that life could be uncertain. That I could let go and "paint a new canvas" in this uncertainty. That beyond a black and white existence, there are more colors to choose from. The journey we make is an inner one. We must come to know ourselves in uncertainty and trust our inner creator and guide.

Your mind is your canvas—paint a masterpiece.

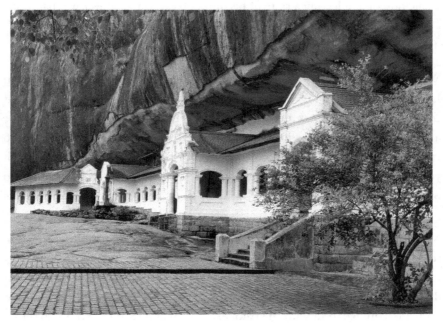

Dambulla Royal Cave Temple and Golden Temple, Sri Lanka, 2019

First, encountering quantum physics was like finding the key (that had been there all along), which unlocked a universe. The pieces fit perfectly. Energy is both a particle and a wave, and our view of it changes that. Think of that! Our view of reality can change the way it flows or becomes what it is. I knew the human mind could create and attract matter and order up the reality that conforms to its view. This means that based on our thoughts, we can be the author of our lives and change the story of our lives. Based on our perspectives and the ability to balance the energies of mind, body, spirit, fuel, and sleep, we can recognize and choose our life's outcomes. Our thoughts, intentions, objects of awareness, conscious actions, and presence with whatever is present impact the results or outcome.

I believe that our existence in this world is for living, living a life full of experiences, based on all the potential inherent in our given lives. Potential experiences can be both attractive and repulsive. We can experience pleasure, pain, suffering, loss, separation, and disappointment in love. We may feel sad and alone, but we are experiencing only feelings, like bubbles in a stream. The bubbles in our bodies, minds, and emotional states are always changing, like a kaleidoscope reflecting a state of becoming based on whatever we manifest.

Tuning into ourselves

When your emotional, physical, or psychological pain is peaking, can you face it without suffering? The first step in solving a problem is to accept that there is a problem. Accepting situations without judging them or feeding the accompanying storyline allows you to get unstuck. Instead of attempting to control your mind, stop and connect with the deepest part of yourself through your breath and calm your mind's chatter. With the breath, you can let go of your mental conditioning and go into your being's microcosm to make different choices.

Mindful moments of self-care and recognition offer us opportunities to weed, seed, and feed virtue, hope, happiness, peace, and freedom from the suffering that catches us in a negative thought process. Our enthusiasm does not depend on things that are external to us. We generate confidence through faith and courage to sit with the pain, examine it and let it go, not by suffering with it. By being present to ourselves with acceptance and awareness, we can be with whatever it is, move into and through feelings, ride them, and be with them without challenging them.

Body, mind, spirit, and connection to a higher power

So how do we get in touch with ourselves? How do we connect with our inner higher power? With every breath, we can practice little habits that help us stay centered and maintain balance while connecting to our emotions and thoughts.

Our bodies, minds, and emotions are integrated and influence each other as a complete unit, which then merges in union with the atmosphere we inhabit. The quote, "A healthy mind is a healthy body" shows an essential part of developing more physical mindfulness, of connecting with spirit and soul. As we encounter different environments, we connect with nature, surrounded by trees, grasses, flowers, soils, water, sky, sun, cold, darkness, and light. We can be better in touch with those vital life forces, the ethereal energies, and the breath of life. We can feel those powers in the trees, the wind, woods, sky, and rich dark soil of the earth, with its nutrients and minerals that feed our souls.

When we are mindful of our thoughts and intentions, especially the negative ones, we need to breathe them in and out. We shift our attention and energies by using compassion and loving-kindness; energy follows attention. When a negative thought emerges, we can recognize it and then nurture it with kindness. We shift our attention elsewhere, removing the weed and seeding it with virtue. Remember, we are the only ones who have power over our bodies, minds, and spirits. Cultivating compassion in our mindfulness and meditation practice shifts our focus to being loving and compassionate and affirms our desire to nurture and create a positive reality.

Techniques and disciplines

Many techniques and holistic disciplines can help us get in touch with ourselves during times of distress. The following are some that I have found beneficial in harmonizing my mind, body, and spirit. It is essential to realize that sorrow, sadness, loss, death, illness, and any other "negative emotions" are not evil. They are all legitimate and must be cared for with compassion and kindness.

These techniques will not circumvent feelings or traumas. They help us navigate life's rough waters and find a safe place inside-out, even while the storm is raging outside.

Mindfulness Meditation

Mindfulness meditation is perhaps the best tool for reconnecting with ourselves and has been covered in previous chapters, but its primary focus is to connect us with our breath. We follow our breath on the inhale and the exhale. Besides getting in touch with ourselves, we can affirm our commitment to being loving and kind. We inhale love and exhale its loss.

Reiki

Reiki is a holistic technique to promote energy balance and self-healing. Among its many benefits, it allows us to bring our mind, body, and spirit into harmony by producing remarkable inner peace. We can practice Reiki on ourselves by being aware of the ethereal (etheric) body and the luminosity of the energy fields surrounding us. These include the physically measurable electromagnetic and magnetic fields generated by all living cells, tissues, and organs within our bodies and biofields, subtle energy bodies, channels, and self-aspects.

Yoga

Yoga is a discipline whose primary purpose is to balance and harmonize our mind, body, and spirit. The different types each have useful characteristics. My primary practice has been integral toga, and over the past twenty-five years, I have had many wonderful energetic benefits in mind, body, and spirit in all aspects of my life.

If you don't feel attracted by a particular discipline, you can always carve out your own daily space (even fifteen to twenty minutes) to relax and meditate in. You can practice meditation with no experience but having a guide to help is highly recommended.

Tune into yourself (meditation)

This psychological technique helps us contact our deep roots, that place inside where our most authentic nature lives. It is an imaginative exercise, a visualization technique, called the Descending Scale Exercise. Do it once a week. Find a quiet place, and memorize the text roughly.

» *Close your eyes and imagine the path inward to that place inside.*

» *Pay attention to your interior, asking yourself,* What is inside me now, right now, in this minute?

» *Open your eyes again. Did you see what it was? Sadness, happiness, bitterness, emptiness, quietness, curiosity, anxiety, anger?*

» *You could also respond with,* Nothing. I'm not feeling anything.

» *Imagine a ladder going down from your head to your heart.*

» *Close your eyes and go back to feeling* what is there now, *but with a difference. Imagine the ladder and go down it into the dark and leave the sensations you were feeling there. Take a step, two steps. Go down for a while and then stop. What is inside you now? Look carefully, feel your state, and open your eyes again.*

» *Listen to your feelings.*

» *What do you experience in your inner world? What is your first feeling or impact? Then descend into the darkness to view what you might refuse to see. Shining a light on it can help you alter your emotional state of being. For some, their restlessness increases and manifests itself as agitation, and for others, feelings of peace come instead.*

» *Find integrity and peace.*

» *Close your eyes and calm your breath. Now focus on your inhalation and exhalation. Then go a little lower, and as you go down, observe what happens inside you. Keep going down, focusing on your breathing until you reach a point where you realize you are at peace.*

» *Try now to go down, narrowing your focus more to a point where a feeling of tranquility, pleasure, or desire arrives, and excitement comes from the dark, the emptiness with no reason or object.*

» *Lose yourself and open your eyes again.*

» *Go down even further until you feel that you have landed in the house of nothing. There is nothing, but it is a nothing in which you expand, in which you lose yourself. Now you can open your eyes.*

Emptiness is form; form is emptiness.

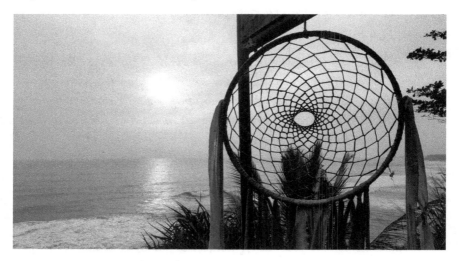

Hot, Little Wind, Ocean, Varkala, Kerala, India, 2019

Meditation helps us to be with our breath and go deep into the chest and stomach. With every breath, we focus on simply being present and aware of mental, emotional, and physical formations. The sky watches the clouds, the rain, the wind and is present for every rotation of the earth's axis. With meditation, we train ourselves to be human beings, not humans doings.

Our brains are meaning-making machines. We need to be watchers of our thought streams to uncover and discover what we are thinking and how it makes us feel. What is present emotionally for you? Is it envy, jealousy, insecurity, aversion, or attraction? What is flowing in the watercourse of your life at this moment, and how are you farming it?

Like farmers who seed, feed, weed, and sow their crops, we need to look at what there is inside of us, accept it, and nurture its growth, or reject it by acknowledging its existence and then letting it go. We don't need to know the cause, and we may not want to know. We don't have to do anything to put things right. We just have to look at the weeds, name them, accept them for what they are, and let them go. We can then plant new seeds of opportunity and potential with our nurturing. They will ripen to life and show up in our lives accordingly.

Fifteen Ways to Connect to Our True Nature

Very often, events carry us away, and emotions blind us to what is around us. We forget to connect to our true nature. What is our true nature? It is the birds, wild animals, air, sun, earth, and water. It is what naturally attracts us in our hearts. In connecting, we let go of deception, the story of who we were or will be "one day," and we let the energy of nature flow through us. We find days turn into nights, weeks into months, and months into years—but are we present to life?

We can be comfortably numb when we operate on autopilot, and our lives are passively submissive to the routine of work, sleep, eat, merely existing so we get by or make it in the world. When we are not awake to the very moment, we miss the sacred moments of truth, where life is incredible.

We live in connection to nature, the rhythms and flows of the day, and the energies that surround us. It interconnects us to the energetic life forces on the planet. When we open to our lives and unplug from the old narratives that have defined us, we can plug into these life-giving energies. It is then refreshing to travel to a new place because we have unplugged from the things and history that previously defined us.

What part of your nature renews and refreshes you?

The following fifteen areas of life may help you unplug from your old ways and plug into a new present moment to connect with your surroundings and nature.

1. Appreciate the people and things present in your life

Sometimes you do not notice the gifts you have until you can no longer have them. Remembering that we all die is one way to get to this point very quickly. You can then cultivate a sense of gratitude for what you have and those who love you and take care of you. Appreciate the people around you and include other people in your life. Celebrate life, and you realize that you have much more than you thought.

2. Stay away from negative people

No one has the right to hurt you or force you to think in a particular way. No one can make you feel inferior, sad, or angry—don't accept the projections of others. Nobody and nothing can ruin your life unless you allow them. You have no control over what others say, but you do have control over their actions. You can decide what you will or won't accept.

3. Cultivate the art of the gift

Forgiveness is a gift that you first give yourself. Forgiving is not about turning the other cheek; it is about letting go of emotional baggage and freeing yourself from the weight of memories, sorrows, and pains. Don't waste time hating people or holding on to memories of people who have hurt you. Wish them love and love the people who love you. When it comes to creating a new story, remember this: the first one who apologizes is the bravest; the first who forgives is the strongest. Be brave. Be strong. Be happy. Be free.

4. Be your authentic self

You, me, and others—we are all unique and extraordinary human beings with one-of-a-kind fingerprints. When you compare yourself with others and despair about your deficiencies, you are doing yourself an injustice. When you believe you need to please everyone and forego your own needs, you compromise your energy. Sometimes you need the courage to be yourself. That may mean that you need to walk away from the people and places that weaken you. You can have the most incredible love affair in life with yourself, your hopes, dreams, and unique energy.

5. Listen to your inner voice

You can't expect to get different results by continuing the same things in the same old way. Listen to your inner voice, the one that guides you and knows where you want to go. It's conscious that you need to listen to your reflective side that provides insight. It's your way and yours alone. If you can find an ally, someone who can walk with you, a mentor or guide, be grateful. Beautiful days give you happiness, and bad days provide experience. The worst days can be the best lessons if you are willing to show up and listen.

6. Break up your routine and embrace change

Remember that you can change the course of your life. It takes one small step every day to change the way you work or cultivate a new hobby. You can try different foods or go to places that you've never been to before. One step a day removes the fear of going back. It lasts a lifetime, and the journey takes only one small step every day.

7. Love yourself and take care of yourself

Loving yourself is the most important thing you can do. When you nurture your soul and take care of your body, you can walk into a relationship with the surrounding world connected with your higher self. When you wake up half an hour earlier in the morning, before others, and greet the new day with gratefulness for the dawn, you can have gratitude for life with a simple smile. Meditate, do yoga, or enjoy breakfast more calmly. Be with yourself and cultivate a relationship of love and acceptance.

8. Love unconditionally

Loving someone does not mean saying "I love you" every day; it means showing it with actions. When you give love, you fill yourself with love. The greatest gift is to be of service. Don't rush love or wait until the "real one" arrives on the scene. Everyone is perfectly imperfect; there is no perfection. On the other hand, do not let loneliness push you into the arms of someone you don't love or someone who doesn't treat you with kindness and respect. When you fall in love, be ready to share your passion and enthusiasm with someone you like to be with. Loving your parents, children, relatives, or friends is a superb way to practice unconditional love. Volunteering and staying close to those who need it are also practical ways to practice "I love you."

9. Remember when you were a child

We were all children once. You can't let your life be too busy or let your mind cloud up with worries. You can't let your heart be closed by old wounds or anger. Imagine that there is a space in your heart where fun, entertainment, and amazement exist. What does that heart space look like? When you allow the child within you to flourish, you learn how to live in the present moment fully. Play with your playful side and live your joy.

10. Spend time with older people

We all get old if we're lucky! Hopefully, you learn something along the way. No one is potentially wiser than those who have already lived most of their lives. They have nothing to lose and everything to remember. Those who have accumulated years, who have overcome obstacles and have managed challenges, have stories and wisdom to tell. Ask them questions. Listen to the advice of those who have lived well. They offer precious knowledge and experience. Give them love and respect, for they are who you will be. Invest in your future, and consider the stories they have created.

11. Focus on what is important to you

You bring about what you think about, so what you focus on matters. Be present with what you are creating or leaving behind at the moment. Time is your most precious commodity. When you wake up, focus on your day. Time never returns. Make a list of four or five things that matter—what is important? Focus on these things and give them time to materialize. Don't delay.

12. Give thanks for problems you don't have

There are two ways to be rich. One is to have everything you want, and the other is to be satisfied with what you have. When you accept and appreciate today's gifts, you will be happier all the time. Happiness comes when you stop complaining about the problems plaguing you and are grateful for those you do not have. We must all fight through some bad days to get to the best ones.

13. Appreciate life's little things

What you appreciate, appreciates in value. The best things in life are free—it's true. Think about it. A sunrise, trees, the ocean, a cool breeze on a hot day, or the sound of a child laughing and playing. It takes very little to be happy, as you watch the sunset on the horizon or spend time with your family. The pandemic of 2020 has provided so many people with a wider perspective—they can enjoy the small things because they realized they were precious. When you adopt the attitude that every day is a blessing, it helps you to see everything as an opportunity to learn, grow, and appreciate the little things in each moment.

14. Accept the past and learn to let go of regrets and future anxieties

Never let your past steal away your present or future. Maybe you aren't proud of everything you've done in the past, but that's okay. The past cannot be changed, forgotten, or canceled. However, you can work through your stories and understand why you did what you did. We all make mistakes, not because we didn't know better, but because we were in pain. You are not your mistakes, and the mistakes you make help define the person you are. You are here, and only you have the power to define who you are and what the future means to you. Some situations or relationships cannot be repaired, and if you insist on fixing them, you may only make the situation worse.

Your actual strength lies in your ability to start all over again. You can have a smile on your face and passion in your heart for what you do. You can forgive, make amends, learn, and grow. You can create the future only by being present to all your possibilities for growth. Never drive forward while looking in the rearview mirror.

15. Get in touch with nature

Go to the mountains, forests, or the beach, away from the concrete jungle of city life and routine. Observe how wonderful and complex the world is and how nature breathes life into each day. When you let yourself be affected by nature's biorhythms, time and space become irrelevant. You can open yourself to the enjoyment and biorhythms of trees, animals, a dark starry night, or the trance of a rainstorm. You can contemplate, let go of your mind and thought processes, allowing yourself to merge with them. You have been lucky enough to see all these natural wonders in this lifetime. Never waste these natural miracles!

Going Inward

In this chapter, we've been looking at how we live in a world on the treadmill of work, acquisition, materialism, and outward appearances. We've also looked at how going inward and living life from the inside-out might seem different for so many. Up until about three hundred years ago, our civilization valued introspection. We thought that reason, wisdom, and the acquisition of knowledge of oneself and the world might help us understand the world better. We looked at the talents of creativity, philosophy, writing, and deep thoughts as rich, fertile ground filled with unexpressed potential.

By going on an inward journey and exploring, we discover our real identities in the world. We connect with our true nature and find possibilities within ourselves—a universe of pure potential. Whatever the mind can conceive or believe, it can achieve. This real universe within is much deeper and more authentic than the external world because it seeds all that materializes in the outer world. Social media, 24/7 news, entertainment, and pop culture mostly demand that we live from the outside-in. Don't listen to that! Turn on your inner light, turn off the world and contemplate, and reflect on your reason for being. Get to know yourself better.

Mindful Tips

Of course, there are no miracles and instant recipes. But there are specific steps we can take to help us know ourselves better as we embark on this journey to spirit and soul.

- Accept yourself for whoever and what you believe yourself to be.
- Recognize the skills and abilities you did not know you had.
- Gain confidence in yourself—you are the only one you've got.
- Transform your limits into strengths and know your limits.
- Be the master of your thoughts and recognize that sometimes it's better not to think.
- Feel comfortable in any situation by accepting yourself in each moment.
- Live every day of your existence at full throttle, at 100 percent, but be sure to apply the brake before around the corners and coast downhill.

By committing yourself to this journey, you will uncover your true self, reconnect with your spirit, and nourish your soul. Most of all, you will grow and connect to yourself and the universe at a deeper level to live the life you want or can imagine.

How do you rate yourself?

Spirit: *Growing and Connecting*

Having a sense of purpose and meaning in your life, feeling connected to something larger than yourself, and finding strength in difficult times.

How do you rate yourself on a scale of 1 (low) to 5 (high)?

Where are you?

1	2	3	4	5

Where do you want to be?

1	2	3	4	5

Why did you choose this number?

What changes could you make to help you get there?

Source: Personal Health Inventory –

Veterans Affairs. https://www.va.gov/WHOLEHEALTH/docs/10-773_PHI_May2020.pdf

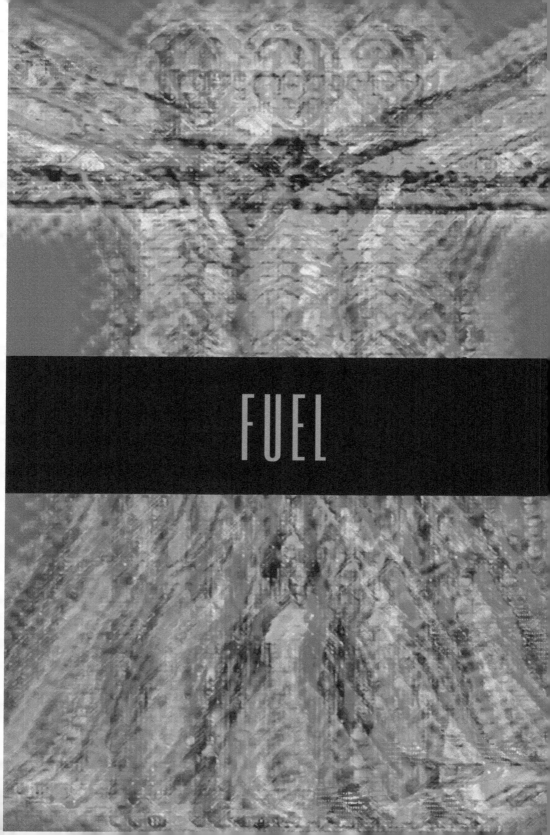

FUEL

Chapter 4

FUEL

Eat and Nourish

FOOD IS THE fuel that powers our bodies and energizes our minds.

There is nothing more important in life than forging exceptional health from food and nourishment. Food is the medicine that feeds, seeds, and weeds our bodies of anything that stops them from growing strong. Food either empowers us or depletes our energy.

Hippocrates's famous saying, "Let food be thy medicine, and let medicine be thy food," is appropriate for this chapter. By looking at our food, we can better understand that we are what we eat.

I am on a 100 percent plant-based diet and am a vigorous advocate for several reasons: overall health, the environment, and nutritional value. I believe that what we eat and drink can nourish our bodies and minds in ways that are foreign to non-plant-based medicines. Whole foods derived from plants and the surrounding wildlife are the most nutritional. If we eat junk, we feel bad and get sick—it's that simple. Choosing a healthy diet and eating habits can be a challenge, given the current, ubiquitous availability of processed and fast food. We have to be diligent, take the supplements that support our health and wellness goals, and limit alcohol, caffeine, and nicotine to keep our bodies and minds healthy. Food is medicine, and medicine is food.

As a two-time cancer survivor, I changed my food habits because I believe that food is the fuel that charges and changes my body's performance. Some people pay more attention to the type of gasoline they put in their cars than the food they put into their bodies. Think about that! If we take care of our bodies with healthy food and nutrition, our bodies will take care of us.

Life is too short to eat terrible food. Our bodies know when they've hit a nasty, worthless piece of food. The sad news is that we will die, but we don't need to hasten that process. Before eating any food, I ask myself, "Will this food nourish my body and mind?" I make a choice. Sometimes it is not the best choice for my body. But I know that, and I consciously choose it anyway. I may not feel happy about it, but I recognize and choose food that helps me create the life I love and the lifestyle I want. The same goes for drinking alcohol or caffeine and taking body- or mind-altering drugs or supplements.

Enter Inside with a Clean Mind and Body

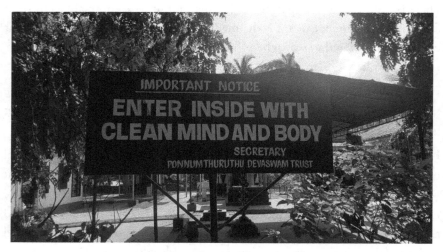

Clean Mind and Body - Anchuthengu, Kerala, India

You might have heard the saying, "The body is a temple." That's an exciting idea to ponder. What do you think it means? I believe it's about how food and nutrition give us life and how food is a sacrament. I don't mean it is part of a religious ceremony, but I believe food is a sacred part of who we are. Food has a mystical role in the evolution of the human race. Evolving from hunter-gatherers to farmers and the Neolithic Age (New Stone Age), humans changed from collected food to producing food. This evolution is perhaps one of the most significant advances in human development. We built permanent shelters. We settled in larger communities and had a broader sense of our abilities to breed, feed, and connect with other human beings. Food was and is an expression of love.

Food gives us energy, information, a sense of connection to each other, and ritual every day. When you think about it, food is the sunshine, the wind, the rain, and the vitamins and minerals that we ingest, digest, and process throughout our bodies. Through it, we commune with the earth, nature, friends, families, and society. Restaurants are the contemporary churches and temples where we meet to celebrate, drink, and eat together. We celebrate birthdays and weddings or go out on our own or with loved ones to eat and commune with others. So, we must get in touch with our food sources and understand how our food is farmed and brought to the market. We must get to know about the way it is prepared and served on our tables. We must take time to savor it and give thanks for what we eat. It is the source of the nutrients we need to live life and thrive.

Scientific studies prove that health comes from the food we eat. It is essential to focus on a varied and balanced diet, that is, a balanced intake of the various nutrients, minerals, and vitamins. Eating is one pleasure of life. However, eating well is not the same as filling up and eating everything on your plate.

Eating healthy food in a friendly environment with people you care for, who care for you, is most important. Grazing on a variety of food is also suitable. As we savor our food, taking the time to eat it, one chew at a time, we can eat less, limiting our intake and enjoying it more. It is a beneficial idea to adopt a food balance routine, not within a single meal or day but preferably over a week, so we have time to look at all foods and balance them in moderation. There are no forbidden foods or miraculous foods. Some are considered healthier, such as fruits, vegetables, whole grains, and fish. Others less so, such as sugary treats, salty foods, red meat, and animal fats. We need to be mindful of our bodies and get a sense of our dietary requirements by having our blood tested for vitamins, minerals, fats, and cholesterol. Bodies have different needs based on their blood type, size, shape, ethnic origin, and temperament.

The benefits of healthy eating

Adopting a suitable eating style helps us build, strengthen, and maintain our bodies. Eating well provides us with the daily energy essential for our bodies to function. Proper nutrition is crucial for healthy physical development throughout life, starting from the prenatal stage. Food and a balanced diet provide for dependable maternal and child health, facilitates child development, and helps adults be more productive. When we don't eat properly, our brains do not get the nutrients required for correct functioning. A brain-boosting diet supports short- and long-term brain function. For example, omega-3 fatty acids help build and repair brain cells, and antioxidants reduce cellular stress and inflammation, linked to brain aging and neurodegenerative disorders, such as Alzheimer's disease.

A balanced diet combined with an active lifestyle, including daily physical activity (chapter 2), helps maintain adequate body weight and promote mind, body, and emotional serenity. Overweight people often tend to be marginalized and subjected to social stigma. Those children develop a problematic relationship with their bodies and peers and consequently isolate themselves even more with an inviting increase in sedentary habits.

Eating healthy helps prevent and treat many chronic diseases, such as obesity, high blood pressure, cardiovascular and metabolic diseases, type 2 diabetes, and some cancers. As a two-time cancer survivor, I am a powerful advocate of food as medicine. A healthy diet strengthens the immune system and helps protect the body from diseases indirectly related to nutrition. I believe that a 100 percent whole food, plant-based diet lifestyle has a direct effect. During challenging times, many people seek foods of poor nutritional value—comfort foods—but they can take a tremendous toll on their bodies, especially when they are vulnerable.

Eating poor nutrient-rich foods

Physiologically, our cardiovascular risks increase with the "wrong" diet. For example, to reduce atherosclerosis and its consequences, it is essential to limit animal fats in our diet. Reducing table salt helps to rebalance blood pressure values and reduce hypertension and heart failure. Meat and animal fats should be reduced to a minimum or eliminated, given their direct link to the risk of tumor development. We are much better off with plant-based whole grains, legumes, or nuts.

Watch out for foods that are heavy in fat, sugar, and salt. An imbalance between caloric intake and energy expenditure combined with a sedentary lifestyle can cause obesity. The World Health Organization defines overweight and obesity as abnormal or excessive accumulation of body fat. Food presents one of the most significant health issues for the American diet today and sadly is why the United States leads the world in obesity.

Eat healthy, nutrient-rich foods

Apply mindfulness to eating well. When we eat by the food's sight, smell, or the taste on our tongue, and its sound, texture, and feel (crunchy, salty, bitter, or sweet), we experience food differently. Taking the time to cook, eat, and share a moment of relaxation are all elements that directly impact our diet, digestion, and weight loss.

Eating healthy and varied

An effective way to ensure an adequate intake of nutrients and energy is to eat various foods. Here are the primary food groups that must be present in our daily diet to ensure we can balance our mind, body, and well-being.

- **Fruits and vegetables:**

  These are fat-free foods rich in vitamins, minerals, and fiber. They have a protective role in the prevention of chronic diseases that appear in adulthood. Be aware of how you eat them. Don't overdo 100 percent pure fruit juices, smoothies, or sauces. Natural sugars in large quantities can be a burden to your liver. Some types of fruit juice or drinks, carbonated drinks, and fruit nectars contain lots of sugar and little fiber. A healthy diet includes at least five portions of fruits and vegetables every day. A portion is the equivalent of about 80 grams (4 grams per teaspoon) of raw fruit or vegetables. It's the amount you can put in the palm of your hand or half a plate of cooked vegetables. You can measure your food using this handful approach to portions—a medium-sized tomato, a handful of cherry tomatoes, a handful of green beans, a bowl of soup, one apple, two apricots, four to five strawberries, or one banana. Eating seasonal fruits and vegetables is always the best approach. It is often cheaper and tastier and filled with more nutrients and vitamins.

- **Starchy foods**

  While most people might move away from starchy foods like cereals, bread, pasta, potatoes, or polenta, consumed moderately daily, they help maintain a balanced diet. They have a high-energy value and do not contain high amounts of fat. Complex grains are better for you. Use light and fat-free dressings and avoid combining foods with lots of butter or sauces. Use the handful approach to limit the use of pasta, bread, or rice, if you do not exercise or burn off carbohydrates quickly or are overweight to obese.

- **Milk and derivatives**

  While their primary function is to supply calcium in a highly absorbable and usable form for your body, I do not believe that dairy products are suitable for the body overall. We get plenty of calcium from vegetables. While calcium is essential for bone construction and maintenance, muscle contraction, and blood clotting, too much of it can create calcium deposits and cardiovascular issues. Use cheeses in moderation and buy them fresh. Don't eat cheeses at the end of a meal. Eat them in moderation, if you must. You can consider cheese as a substitute for meat or fish. Do your best to limit all dairy products.

- **Fish, meat, eggs, soy, and beans**

  These foods provide you with protein. Meat and fish provide iron. Fish also has a protective effect because of omega-3 fatty acids, which reduce cardiovascular disease risk. You can eat meat, fish, or eggs, but limit your overall consumption. As for fish, eat it (both fresh and frozen) at least two times a week. Lean meats (chicken and turkey) are fine, too, if you must. I prefer soy and beans of all kinds, such as peas, chickpeas, and lentils. They are a marvelous addition to your diet. New meat substitutes offer meat eaters practical alternatives, as they have attractive textures and add tasty flavors to meals. The other options are usually cheaper than meat and fish but are just as nutritious, giving us iron, fiber, vitamins, and minerals. With the new alternative options, grilling still works. Whatever you choose, limit your use of fat-rich sauces and fatty foods.

- **Condiment fats**

  Limit the use of fatty oils or butter. Use extra virgin olive oil sparingly, rather than vegetable oils. Limit or eliminate animal fats, such as butter, lard, cream, or any saturated fats. Excessive fat consumption increases the risk of being overweight and the development of calcium deposits in the arteries, or the heart, leading to cardiovascular diseases. Remember that oils have a high-energy value, and hidden fats are already present from the manufacturing process. Stay as natural and whole to the food source as you can.

Additional food insights for mindful eating

- Do your best to eliminate salt from your diet. Excessive consumption can cause moderate-to-severe hypertension and cardiovascular disease. Remove or reduce salt during cooking and add more spice and aromatic herbs. Pay attention to the salt in packaged foods. Remember that four grams of salt equal one teaspoon. I am amazed at how much salt we add to "natural foods."

- Enjoy sweet foods and beverages in moderation because they are rich in fats and sugars are highly caloric and fatty and can lead to diabetes and other cardiovascular and pulmonary complications.

- Top off your meals with fruit or homemade desserts with reduced sugar. The rule of thumb is to taste everything mindfully and savor the food; roll it around your tongue and lips. Eat to taste.

Drink water in large quantities because our bodies comprise over 60 percent water, though we lose a part of it through sweat, urine, and breathing (respiration). To stay physically fit, drink 50 percent of your body weight in ounces. Don't wait until you feel thirsty before you drink—your body will already be short of water. Water is vital in hot weather and particularly for children and the elderly. If you have difficulty drinking plain water, prepare an herbal tea or an infusion or flavor the water with a few mint leaves, lemon juice, or a slice of orange.

Savor everything you eat and drink. Think about your choices. Why do you eat? Think about the times of day and times you eat, rather than when you are hungry. Consider what you eat. Is it healthy for you? Will the food give you energy or take it away? Think about how you eat. Is it quickly or slowly? Do you taste the food or shovel it down? How much do you eat? Do you eat until you are full, or do you leave room for digestion? Where do you eat? Do you take the time to create a ritual around the food that is going into your body? Make your choices mindful by planning, selecting, and savoring what you eat.

Inflammation: Foundation of Everything

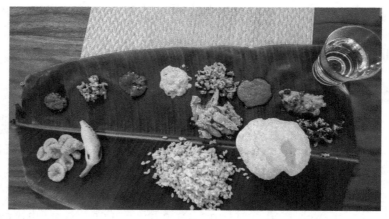

Mekosha, Ayurvedic Retreat, Keezhattingal, Kerala, India, 2019

Scientific research has discovered that the basis of degenerative diseases lies in our relationship with inflammation. Arthritis, diabetes, Alzheimer's disease, osteoporosis, acne, psoriasis, tumors, skin aging, and wrinkles are related to inflammation, increasing with aging.

Inflammation is necessary and is a vital part of the immune system's response to injury and infection. Chemically, it is the body's way of signaling the immune system to heal and repair damaged tissue and defend itself against viruses, bacteria, and other foreign invaders. The inflammation process enables our bodies to respond to wounds that might otherwise fester and become infected and potentially deadly.

A healthy diet and lifestyle can help keep inflammation under control. Authentic nutrition enables us to move into our daily tussle and flow with life. With adequate nutrition from minerals, vitamins, and nutrients, our bodies are better equipped. Eating well includes drinking enough water to oxidize and eliminate toxins. Getting up and moving our bodies helps us to tone and tighten our bodies as well.

What is the food inflammation index?

Due to their characteristics, foods can be pro-inflammatory, anti-inflammatory, or neutral, which we know as highly acidic, alkaline, or neutral.

Pro-inflammatory foods can worsen the state of inflammation. They are the "industrial foods" that are processed and contain saturated fats, cholesterol, additives, dyes, sweeteners, and flavor enhancers:

- Industrial sweets and snacks
- Ready-made soups
- Ready-made sauces
- Processed meats
- Cold cuts (saturated fat and cholesterol)
- Sausages
- Breaded chicken and fish fillets
- Alcohol
- Potatoes and chips

In general, **anti-inflammatory foods** are of vegetable origin and are rich in fiber and micronutrients:

- Cereals, particularly whole grain, wheat, rice, oats, barley, spelt, rye, buckwheat, and millet

- Extra virgin olive oil (monounsaturated fats, vitamin E, and polyphenols)

- Onions

- Apples

- Flax and pumpkin seeds

- Almonds and walnuts

- Berries

- Turmeric and ginger

- Pineapple

I prefer anti-inflammatory foods with a low inflammation index. They have helped me deal with cardiovascular disease, weight gain, and degenerative conditions.

The inflammatory food index may be a novelty to many. The theory adds little to the natural health and wellness experience. For health and wellness, consume more whole grains, extra virgin olive oil, eat five portions of fresh vegetables and fruit a day, drink lots of water, some dried fruit (almonds, nuts), and limit all industrially processed foods. Industrially prepared foods require no or minimal domestic preparation, each one of them is a source of processed and refined sugars that can lead to obesity in the long term.

Choosing the Right Foods

Healthy foods help us develop healthier bodies and overcome anxiety, stress, and physical ailments. Many studies have shown that eating can be more effective than drugs in nourishing us on the road to wellness. Healthy eating helps us prevent and cure many diseases, and it promotes mental and physical well-being.

Some foods can ease and often resolve small and large disorders that negatively affect our lives (from insomnia to constipation). They make us feel more energetic and vital, or they protect us from stress, tension, and nervousness.

You must choose the right foods and stay away from those that can hurt your mental and physical balance. Do not think of nutritious food as a medicine to be taken only when an illness starts. Think of food as a lifestyle choice, a source of energy that strengthens your mind, body, and spirit every day.

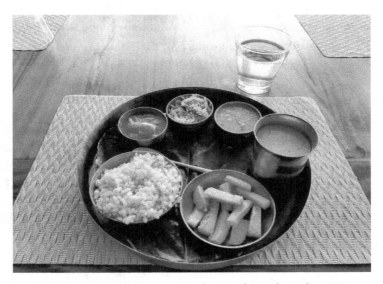

Mekosha, Ayurvedic Retreat, Keezhattingal, Kerala, India, 2019

The best foods align with your body type. Look at and explore Ayurvedic diets and the idea of having a specific dosha (energy system) that aligns with your body type. You can find plenty of information on the web to take a dosha quiz to assess if you have a Vata, Pitta, or Kapha body type. Your dosha has many corresponding qualities expressed in physical, emotional, and mental aspects. We all have elements of each dosha, but one or two doshas tend to dominate. Do your best to eat foods that you have an interest in that also pay dividends.

Foods that do not pay rent

Junk food is high in calories and negatively affects your body, emotions, and overall psychological well-being. A study published in the *Public Health Nutrition* journal showed that those who regularly consume snacks, cheeseburgers, and hot dogs are more likely to develop depressive states (+51 percent).[11]

---

11 https://www.sciencedaily.com/releases/2012/03/120330081352.htm

People still eat junk food. Why? Chemically engineered junk food triggers dopamine production in the body to provide a momentary physical and mental rush. Animal fats, chemicals, and refined sugars activate cortisol, the stress hormone, causing a glycemic swell. When the blood sugar level reduces again, it can cause an emotional breakdown, anxiety, depression, stress, fatigue in adults, and distraction and hyperactivity in children. I believe the science.

Eye to coffee

Coffee stimulates adrenaline production, the hormone of fear, which helps to trigger states of anxiety and agitation. The ideal is not to exceed one or two cups a day. Eliminate coffee and replace it with boiling water and lemon or tea in the morning. Doing that helps digestion, the caffeine rush is not as intense, and your emotional state will be calmer.

Foods that pay rent

Foods that "pay rent" have various benefits to your mind, body, and emotional balance. By eating right for you, you can boost your mood and temperament.

Research conducted on nearly three hundred young people around the age of twenty, from the New Zealand University of Otago, revealed the positive effects of eating fruits and vegetables. The kids who ate more fruits and vegetables during the day said they felt calmer, happier, and more energetic than usual. A study by the University of Warwick confirmed these results. They observed the eating habits of 80,000 people in Britain. The researchers discovered that those who consumed fruits and vegetables every day felt more peaceful than others and even happier if they ate seven servings a day. [12]

Fruits and vegetables are rich in folic acid (contained in spinach, asparagus, oranges, juices, and legumes) and other minerals and vitamins that help regulate serotonin levels. Serotonin helps you to manage your emotions and keep your emotional balance. So, bump up your intake of fruits and vegetables every day. Have up to five servings a day for your health, physical fitness, mood, and emotional well-being.

---

12 https://www.sciencedaily.com/releases/2020/12/201216094647.htm

Vitamin D

The natural source of vitamin D is the sun from being outdoors in natural landscapes. Getting enough vitamin D is one of the most significant issues most people have with maintaining their health. Food rich in vitamin D will help you combat stress and metabolize and store calcium in your body. Vitamin D deficiency can impact mood, depression, and anxiety. Eating foods like egg yolks, cheese, cod liver oil, beef, liver, and fatty fish like tuna, salmon, sardines, herring, and mackerel have relatively low levels of Vitamin D. The best sources for Vitamin D can be found outdoors, near rivers, mountains, streams, lakes, or oceans—walking in the sunshine. It is indeed the most significant source of life.

Regain energy with vitamin B_{12}

Sadness is often a consequence of being fatigued. You could also be weak and not very quick, physically or mentally. Are you getting enough B_{12} in your diet? B_{12} boosts your energy and calms your nerves for maintaining a healthy, stressless perspective.

It is one vitamin that many vegetarians miss because it's in many animal foods, like meat, fish, and dairy products. Clams, mussels, mackerel, herring, and animal liver are great sources for B_{12}.

If you have a vitamin B_{12} deficiency, you might experience anemia or issues with your nervous system. Vegan sources of B_{12} are foods fortified with B_{12}, including plant milk, soy products, breakfast cereals, and B_{12} supplements. Whether in supplements, fortified foods, or animal products, Vitamin B_{12} comes from microorganisms.

Omega-3s—essential for our well-being

Omega-3s have many powerful health benefits for our bodies and brains. Omega-3s are in the various membranes surrounding our neurons throughout our bodies. They act as signaling points between the brain and the multiple cells that guide our bodies to receive nutrients. A diet rich in omega-3 fatty acids helps us have a younger, more energetic brain with more vital cognitive abilities. Omega-3s act as a shield against the adverse effects of free radicals by acting as antioxidants. Omega-3 improves heart and eye health. It reduces

ADHD symptoms in children, helps metabolic syndrome, fights inflammation and autoimmune disease, improves mental disorders, fights age-related Alzheimer's, helps prevent cancer, and reduces fat in our liver—and has other benefits as well.

Omega-3s are effective against depression. These fatty acids help us to smile more and give us quicker minds. Eating healthy foods like salmon, sardines, trout, mackerel, and tuna is sufficient for most. But we vegetarians and vegans need to add seaweed, nori, spirulina, and chlorella. Seaweed and algae are important sources of omega-3 because they are one of the few plant groups that contain DHA and EPA.

Don't forget the minerals

Finally, to cheer you up and find momentum on the darkest days, fill up with minerals! Magnesium, zinc, selenium, and potassium are in abundance in dried fruit, and these minerals give you energy, fight fatigue, keep insomnia away, and relieve a lousy mood—one disorder of the classic premenstrual syndrome.

Worthwhile magnesium sources are whole wheat, spinach, quinoa, almonds, cashews, peanuts, dark chocolate (my favorite), black beans, edamame, and avocado.

The Psychology of Good Food

How serotonin affects psychological well-being

We are in a lousy mood, triggered, and emotionally hi-jacked. How is it that we want to eat chocolate when we are in a grim mood? Why do we want to cuddle with a glass of milk and cookies? Why do women feel the need to eat sweets during their menstrual cycle?

There are scientific answers to all these questions. Our bodies produce a substance called serotonin, which focuses on the psychology of well-being.

Serotonin is an important chemical and neurotransmitter in the human body. Science shows that it helps regulate mood and social behavior, appetite, digestion, sleep, memory, and sexual desire and function. Serotonin stimulates feelings of pleasure, calm, and relaxation. Chocolate is a food that promotes serotonin production and improves our psychological well-being. It contains

other substances that produce endorphins, contributing to the body's ability to rest and relax. The same is true for milk and honey. Serotonin has a fundamental role in controlling appetite and eating behavior.

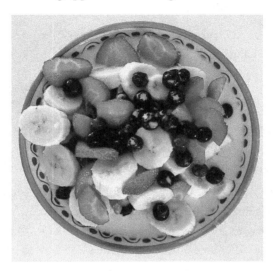

Yummy dessert for breakfast, fresh fruits, nuts, almond milk, 2019

Serotonin helps the body to feel a sense of satiety and control the need to eat food. It is also known as the good mood hormone. When people suffer from eating disorders and mood declines, they often take medicines that increase the need for serotonin. It also intervenes to help blood pressure and the contraction of arteries, bronchi, bladder, intracranial vessels, and smooth muscles. It works on our parasympathetic nervous systems, allowing us to rest and digest.

Some studies have shown associations between low serotonin levels and aggressive behavior, anxiety, depression, insomnia, irritability, poor appetite, social anxiety, panic disorders, poor memory, and more. Foods that increase the serotonin levels in our body are:

- Eggs
- Salmon
- Pineapple
- Cheese

- Tofu

- Nuts and Seeds

- Turkey (tryptophan)

Food and supplements aren't the only ways to boost serotonin levels. We can also look at daily habits for increasing our levels and for getting fit.

- **Exercise.** Having regular exercise can have antidepressant effects and help boost serotonin.

- **Sunshine**. Being exposed to bright light boosts serotonin levels. Getting outdoors helps us sleep better, too, so try it and take a walk outside during lunch or when your mind is wandering.

- **Positive Attitudes**. Our bodies respond to positivity. Having a sense of gratitude lifts our attitude and boosts our serotonin levels. Learn how to smile even if you don't feel like it. Our bodies don't know the difference and respond the same way to both.

- **Cultivate Gut Bacteria**. A high-fiber diet helps to fuel healthy gut bacteria, which plays a role in serotonin levels. Check out supplemental probiotics, lemon juice, apple cider vinegar (my favorite), and pickled foods too.

Which foods to prefer

British researchers of the Food and Mood Project Association conducted a study for 5 years of 550 people with depression.[13] After carefully following all the nutritionists' advice, about 88 percent of patients said they felt better, while 26 percent reported a reduction in their mood swings.

Dairy products, potatoes, pumpkins, figs, and bananas are fine, but coffee and alcohol mask fatigue and even destroy essential vitamins needed for psychological and physical well-being. Nutrition and mental well-being are closely related.

---

13   http://news.bbc.co.uk/2/hi/health/2264529.stm

Psychological well-being

By cultivating a practice of mindfulness while eating, sleeping, walking, and being with others, we can generate an increased sense of well-being. We can develop a sense of belonging. When we communicate and connect with others, face-to-face or virtually, we have a more refined understanding of ourselves. We see ourselves as others see us for our contribution. We see others, and they see us as well. As we come to understand others, we have an expanded sense of gratitude. A sense of being self-directed is essential.

Sleep and diet

Food and energy directly depend on sleep. Overall, people who are sleep deprived tend to weigh more and have more trouble losing weight than those who get adequate rest even when they follow the same diet. When we don't get enough sleep, our bodies overproduce the hormone ghrelin, which handles hunger and appetite and plays a role in weight gain. We generate ghrelin during the night, increasing the desire for sweets and carbohydrates during the other hours of the day. So, do your best to get a good night's sleep as part of your daily routine if you want to avoid excessive weight gain.

Satiety also depends on the amount of leptin in the blood; insomniacs don't have enough of this hormone in their bodies. Fat cells make leptin, which decreases your appetite. When we get enough sleep, our bodies naturally produce it.

Diet tips for better sleep

When we sleep better, we eat less and take off extra pounds. By avoiding foods with excessive sodium content, such as pretzels and potato chips, we sleep better. When we focus on foods that help us relax our bodies, like rice, pasta, bread, barley, or foods containing the amino acid tryptophan, we sleep better. These foods facilitate the synthesis of serotonin, the hormone that stimulates the relaxation response. We should reduce our intake of meats, fish, or cheese to help with digestion. In my 100 percent plant-based diet, I do not eat any dairy, meat, fish, or animal products.

Do your research to see what specific role foods have in promoting sleep. Everybody is different, and you've got to find out how particular foods react to your body.

Five Health Benefits of Plant-Based Diets

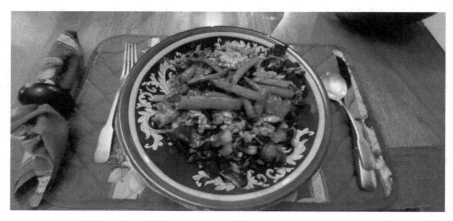

Plant-based dinners are great fun to make at home, 2017

So, do we do fat-free, sugar-free, or gluten-free? What to do? Fortunately, there is a diet model that doctors, nutritionists, and scientists generally agree on for its ability to help prevent disease and even prolong life. This diet, which is naturally rich in fiber, nutrients, and antioxidants, is plant based.

A plant-based diet is based more on plant sources, such as fruits, vegetables, and whole grains, rather than animal sources, such as meat and dairy products.

A plant-based diet can start with a vegan approach, which excludes all animal products, including eggs and dairy products. A vegetarian plant-based diet excludes meat, poultry, and fish products but includes eggs and dairy. Other options are possible, such as adding fish but still excluding meat and poultry. If you go with a 100 percent plant-based diet, you'd opt for more of a vegan diet, a healthy challenge, but well worth it in so many ways.

I went to a 100 percent plant-based diet, so I am getting a diet rich in fruit, vegetables, whole grains, nuts, legumes, soy, and no dairy. Add a minimal amount of meat, dairy products, eggs, and refined foods based on how you feel. Author Michael Pollan summarized the power of plants in his book, *In Defense of Food: An Eater's Manifesto*, in seven simple words, "Eat food. Not too much. Mainly plants."[14]

---

14   https://michaelpollan.com/books/in-defense-of-food/

Five key benefits

Plant-based nutrition is not a new trend; it's been around for centuries, and that is part of how we know it has such dramatic health benefits. Studies have found that some populations living in the Mediterranean have a significantly lower risk of cancer than those living in the United States and Northern Europe. Researchers have attributed this to their eating habits. The Mediterranean diet, rich in fruits and vegetables and low in red meat, has an incredibly protective effect on the body. As a two-time cancer survivor, I attribute much of my good health to a predominantly plant-based diet. Here are five sound reasons for looking at incorporating more plants into your diet.

1. Prevent chronic diseases

It turns out an apple a day keeps the doctor away. A diet rich in fruits and vegetables can help prevent chronic diseases. Many studies have linked plant-based diets to protecting the body from cancer and diabetes.

Why? A plant-based diet is naturally low in saturated fat, high in fiber, and lower in added sugars. More than diets that include animal food and processed foods, a plant-based diet keeps you healthy. It can also help you lose weight, improve your blood sugar, and lower your blood pressure.

The comforting news is that you can start small and still see some significant changes. A 2016 study published in *PLOS Medicine* found that even minor changes to your diet can help lower your risk of diabetes. They linked cutting daily portions of animal products from 6 to 4 servings to a lower incidence of diabetes. [15]

Studies have also shown that even if you have diabetes, adhering to a plant-based diet can help reverse the disease and improve your blood sugar.

2. Improve your mood

Besides reducing the risk of cancer and diabetes, a diet rich in plant-based foods can increase your happiness levels, according to studies. That makes me happy!

---

15   https://journals.plos.org/plosmedicine/article?id=10.1371/journal.pmed.1002700

While we all know that eating berries and broccoli benefits your long-term physical health, it is also helpful for your mental well-being. A 2016 study by the *American Journal of Public Health* found that increasing fruits and vegetable consumption over two years was "equal in size to the psychological gain resulting from the transition from unemployment to employment."[16] How? A plant-based diet provides the antioxidants to fight inflammation and the phytochemicals to regulate the brain's chemicals that control mood. That's why green is excellent for us too.

3. Protect your heart

Helping your heart with fruits, vegetables, and whole grains means that you can live longer. Eating a plant-based diet can lower your blood pressure and reduce the risk of heart disease by up to a third.

Studies found that a diet rich in vegetables can deactivate specific genes, making them less susceptible to heart disease. It seems incredible, but such is the power of plants. Looking to epigenetics—the science of how our lifestyles interact with our genes—studies have found that we can change our genes for the better when we make lifestyle changes and incorporate a plant-based diet into our daily routine.

4. Get rid of excess weight

Say goodbye to calorie counting and deceptive diets. A plant-based diet does not require special tools or tricks, only fresh products, cereals, and legumes. The probability of losing a couple of pounds is an attractive proposition to many. It's not magic; it's all about digestion and elimination.

A study published in the *Journal of the Academy of Nutrition and Dietetics* evaluated 15 different plant-based diets and found that, on average, participants lost about 7.4 pounds (which includes those who did not stick to the diets).[17] The high-fiber content in a plant-based diet can lead to feelings of satiety, which helps with weight loss.

---

16   https://www.ncbi.nlm.nih.gov/pmc/articles/PMC4940663/

17   https://www.ncbi.nlm.nih.gov/books/NBK278991/

5. Longevity and energy

Kale, yes! Those who follow a plant-based diet can live a longer life. Studies show that plant-based diets are associated with a lower risk of death, and a Mediterranean-type diet increases the telomere length of our DNA. These DNA–binding protein structures, found at both ends of each chromosome, protect the genome from degradation. The better the lifestyle and numbers of plants, the longer the telomeres and the lifespan.

Mindful eating involves being awake and alive to a better lifestyle and eating, feeding the body with nutrients and food that benefit us nutritionally and have definite lifestyle benefits. It is clear that recognizing nutritious food and making healthy choices help us to live healthier and longer. What we eat, how we sleep, how physical and active we are, and what we expose ourselves to—like smoking, excessive alcohol consumption, or other toxic substances—contributes to our overall health.

Mindful Tips

This chapter has outlined multiple food options for integrating into our lives and lifestyles. You don't need to make drastic changes overnight, but you would be wise to make them gradually and use "compassionate discipline" to make them stick. You can make a difference in your life and the lives of others, but it takes a mindful approach and a choice to do so. Ask yourself before you eat, What does my body need? How can I treat my body well? What can I eat that will help me eliminate the negative and stress the positive?

According to the latest estimates, 800 million people worldwide are over the age of 60, and by 2050 there will be about two billion of them. Advances in healthcare and nutrition will help us live healthier lifestyles. With the proper education, we can make a difference, shift our perspectives about food, and respect our bodies and minds.

How do you rate yourself?

Fuel: Eat and Nourish.

I am eating healthy, balanced meals with plenty of fruits and vegetables each day, drinking enough water, and limiting sodas, sweetened drinks, and alcohol.

How do you rate yourself on a scale of 1 (low) to 5 (high)?

Where are you?

1	2	3	4	5

Where do you want to be?

1	2	3	4	5

Why did you choose this number?

_____

_____

_____

What changes could you make to help you get there?

_____

_____

_____

Source: Personal Health Inventory –

Veterans Affairs. https://www.va.gov/WHOLEHEALTH/docs/10-773_PHI_May2020.pdf

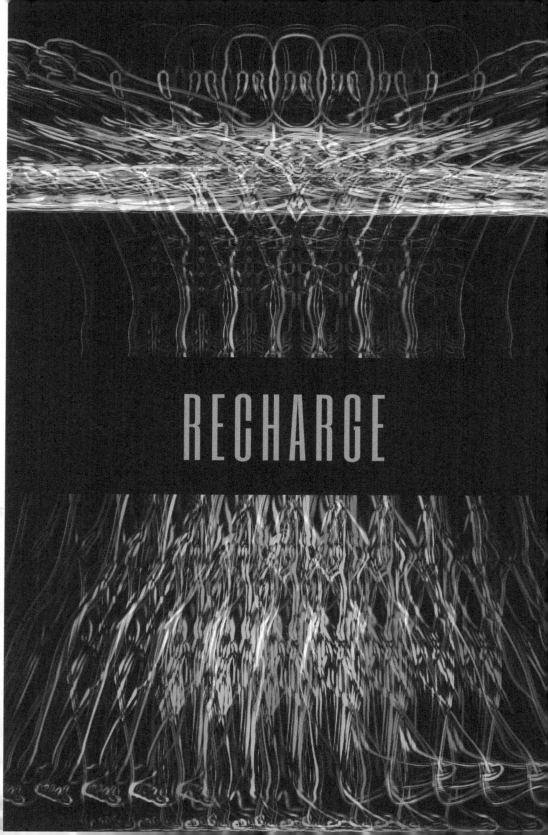

RECHARGE

Chapter 5
RECHARGE

Sleep and Refresh

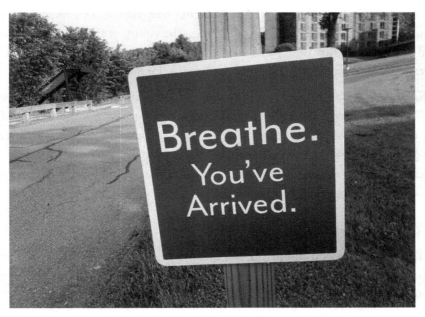

Welcome sign, Kripalu Retreat and Yoga Center, 2018

SLEEP IS ESSENTIAL for our bodies, minds, and spirits. The Dalai Lama knows the importance of sleep. In 1989, he said, "Sleep is the best meditation."[18]

---

18   https://shugdensociety.wordpress.com/2009/11/05/
evidence-of-deception-in-the-dalai-lamas-own-words/

The most recent studies reveal that sleep patterns allow the brain to clean the waste accumulated while we are awake. Rest can give us peace and relaxation, lower stress, help us feel recharged and refreshed, and ground us with a more transparent, clearer perspective on life. The right balance between activity and rest improves our health and well-being. This chapter looks at how to sleep. A minimum of seven hours a day can revitalize us to live a more mindful life.

While sleep is an essential part of who we are and a necessary part of a healthy body and mind, we can often get lost in crazy routines and busy lifestyles that busy our minds and keep us up. We can miss a good night's sleep because of work worry, responsibilities, and planning, which creep into a restful sleep. With too much rumination, we sleep less and may even have insomnia, which results in diminished concentration and focus during the day. We may experience memory loss and be disconnected, distracted, and not engaged—commonly known as brain fog. A poor night's sleep significantly impacts brain function. Sleep is vital for brain plasticity—the ability of the brain to process and adapt to inputs. It is critical to the brain's ability to learn, grow, and integrate so that we can remember and access it in the future.

When we mindfully sleep and recharge, we get ourselves prepared for bed. We plant the seeds for sound, restful sleep, setting in place the causes and conditions that make it so. Our sleep helps to fight the formation of free radicals, the aging process, and various degenerative diseases, including cancer, dementia, and coronary problems. It is beneficial to let go of our devices and to-do lists and get ready to take a flight to dreamland.

Tips for more and better sleep

Changing habits and improving the quality of life depends on each person's choices. Here are some rules and simple tips to improve the quality of your sleep.

- Reduce daily stress.
- Maintain a varied and balanced diet, preferably of plant-based organic foods.
- Practice physical activity regularly (preferably once a day for thirty to sixty minutes).

- Respect moments of relaxing breaks and leisure—you don't live to work.

- Set healthy limits for your personal and professional life.

- Take time for a hobby or an activity that promotes psychophysical balance, such as yoga or Pilates.

And finally, don't underestimate the importance of consulting with a sleep disorder specialist. The doctor will evaluate the need to start a treatment based on homeopathic or pharmacological products to reduce stress and help you sleep better.

Healthy living requires a fair amount of physical activity, a balanced diet, and rest. These three elements are all critical. All are equally fundamental, and we need to make the sacrifices, but for quality of life, it is worth it. One way of getting the necessary balance is to divide the hours of a twenty-four-hour day by the things you want to do. One day has twenty-four hours; ideally, eight are for work, seven are for sleeping, and the remaining nine are for what you like to do! If you don't know what you want, then get busy. Life is passing by, and you've got to be a part of it. Wake up!

The Importance of Relaxation

Work takes up most of our time in adult life and significantly affects our level of well-being. If we lose a night's sleep, there are serious consequences. If we regularly work for sixteen hours and sleep four hours a night, we pay a high price. We can become completely absorbed by work, continually doing more, and not leave enough time for the body to eliminate the toxins it accumulates. Our livers and kidneys need time to complete their daily cleansing process. When that doesn't happen, fatigue sets in, and our days are even more challenging.

When we are fresh and rested, we can count on our bodies and minds to support us in making rational decisions when we communicate and connect with others. Activities are more manageable when we are more open and receptive. We must be consistent and do our best to rest at a regular interval. Maintaining the rigor of our activities and focusing on rest, exercise, and work allows us to develop healthier minds, bodies, and spirits.

Why is it so difficult to rest enough?

More than once, you may have heard someone say, "There is not enough time in a day to do what I need to do!" Indeed, many people stress because there is too much to do. But think of our parents or grandparents. They didn't have the convenience of dishwashers, microwaves, or programmable devices to help them get more out of their day. We have technology everywhere and everything at our fingertips, including stores selling cooked food. But times have changed, life's rhythm is stressful, and trauma has increased since the beginning of COVID. Our priorities and stressors push away our sense of balance, and we forget to get enough rest.

Why is it important to get enough rest?

Energy recovery

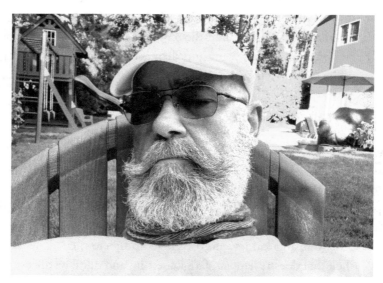

A summer afternoon nap, during Covid pandemic, 2020

We all exert energy and exert even more when we worry. When we sleep, we allow our organs to rest and recover all the energy consumed. After an exhausting day, our bodies are ready to reboot, and we reboot and recharge. When we sleep, we prepare to face another busy day.

Cortisol

Stress activates the production of cortisol in the body, and if it is not used or attended to correctly, people will undoubtedly suffer from a lack of sleep. They will be too alert and ready for whatever disaster—real or imagined—awaits them. It can also produce other unpleasant symptoms, such as hair loss, crusting on the head, skin lesions, and excessive tiredness.

Mood swings

Without sufficient rest, our mood suffers. We experience abrupt changes of spirit, which lead to problems in our families, work environments, and friendships. If we are down, we can view life with a lot of negativity, which further escalates our relationships and physical or emotional health.

Increased body weight

Not sleeping or resting enough creates hormonal and metabolic imbalances that lead to weight gain. Even if we make sacrifices, follow a healthy lifestyle, and play sports, that commitment will be useless if we do not rest adequately. When we don't sleep well, the body's adrenal glands produce cortisol, which triggers the release of glucose. A rush of glucose raises insulin levels. Cortisol prompts the body to store fat (primarily in the abdomen) as a backup fuel source. Abdominal fat and obesity are linked to chronic elevations of cortisol in many studies. Being overweight translates into risk factors for diseases, such as diabetes, hypertension, and other cardiovascular disorders.

Sleep builds resilience

Getting a good night's sleep helps us overcome physical, cognitive, and emotional imbalances more easily. The research is detailed, showing that those who suffer from sleep disorders are more likely to develop depression, anxiety, stress, or anger. Thus, sleeping well helps prevent many ailments.

Sleep is also essential for reducing the constant feeling of tiredness and improving our health. By sleeping adequately, we can speed up our metabolisms and achieve a higher degree of performance professionally and personally.

Sleep increases physical endurance

Our bodies need to regain strength before facing another day. If our day is full of commitments, challenges, and challenging emotions, sleep directly affects us on a cellular level and impacts our metabolism, our immune system, and our ability to respond effectively. People who sleep well and rest are more resistant to pain and illness.

Sleeping well decreases the risk of Alzheimer's

Recent studies have identified an increased concentration of Alzheimer's biomarkers in people who slept less than five hours a day. Likewise, those who slept six to eight hours a day but had sleep disorders had the same biomarkers. That is something to consider.

The Importance of Rest after Physical Exercise

Balance your rest and physical activity if you want to feel better. Training and challenging physical limits are essential for any athlete, and rest is equally important. Many athletes underestimate or forget the importance of rest, resulting in fatigue, poor performance, and injury.

Rest is an essential part of the various training components—between different exercises, between one training session and another (for example, morning and afternoon), and between the week's days.

The general recommendation for those who practice amateur sports is to avoid training for a minimum of two days a week, preferably three. This timing can vary for professionals and athletes at a competitive level because coaches generally create a particular program of complementary exercises that vary in intensity and allow them to exercise different muscles and abilities every day.

Muscle recovery

For training, the body requires a higher level of functioning than usual. It is necessary, therefore, to allow the body to return to its normal activity levels afterward.

During the sleep process, our bodies are recharged and restored with glycogen, a vital substance that can be converted into glucose when the muscles require energy.

Increased muscle mass

When training, working with weights can damage the fibers and tissues that make up our muscles. Damage is repaired during periods of inactivity and sleep with the help of our dietary proteins. These regenerative muscle processes occur during sleep, and a good night's rest helps us develop and grow muscle.

Rest for the mind

No matter how passionate you are about sports, there is always a time when you need to stop and take a break. During training sessions and competitions, your mind is under pressure from the effort required to succeed.

Avoid burnout

You cannot train or exercise every day. Your mind and body need rest too. If not, you become demotivated, your performance suffers. You will experience loss and failure, and you won't achieve your objectives. Burnout occurs at home, at work, and can also happen in the sporting context.

What happens when we don't rest?

Many athletes report a drop in performance after one or more days of rest, but there is no evidence to support that claim. The evidence shows that we require two weeks of inactivity to experience a significant drop in performance. In all kinds of sports, professional teams have at least one day off during the week, particularly after a competition or the day after that.

Injuries

In most cases, excessive training causes cramps, contractures (muscle tightening), and muscle fiber injuries. An athlete can face a mandatory two- or three-week break in the worst case by avoiding one or two days off.

Not respecting rest days can cause stress injuries. Subject the joints or bones to steady pressure, movement, or impact, and injuries occur. In the long run, the lack of rest causes severe damage to the body, including bone fractures.

Demotivation and failure to achieve results

Rest is essential if the changes that occur after the body's physical effort are to provide resilience. If we don't rest, we experience a decrease in performance.

A decrease in performance caused by fatigue—even moderate fatigue—leads to a state of demotivation. It's essential to take the time to be mindful and feed the mind, body, and spirit, and even consider a day off as one for "passive training" so we can recharge our batteries. On these days, it is beneficial to maintain proper nutrition and relax the mind with recreational activities that do not require excessive physical effort.

When you are always on the move, it's easy to forget what natural relaxation is and how to reach it and feel rested. You can feel overwhelmed by a kind of frustration that will lead you to think you are incapable of pulling the plug. Some people find it more beneficial to watch a horror movie than to lie on a beach with the sea's sound in the background. I've tried both and often find that resting on the couch with a good movie is enough. Although, as I write this, I am in my backyard, listening to the birds and enjoying a cool breeze while I'm working. So, there are exceptions.

There is no single universally recognized way to relax. The means and tools change from person to person, so find your way to deal with daily stresses in your personal life and workplace.

The Best Ways for Mindful Recharging

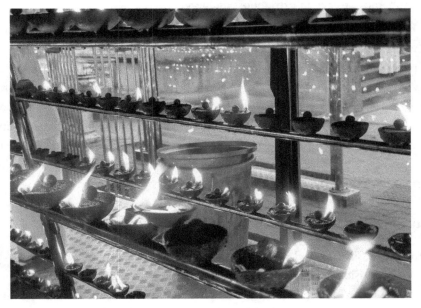

Candle lighting ceremony, Sri Lanka Pilgrimage, 2019

I have found that if simple rest does not help me recover from fatigue caused by stress or excessive working hours, I can find relief, generate energy, and even relax with some simple remedies.

Aromatherapy—I like to moisten a tissue with a drop of rosemary, peppermint, or basil on it. Smelling the aroma guarantees me a burst of energy. Even pouring ten drops of rosemary on a washcloth or in the bathwater can restore me to alertness in a few minutes.

Hydrotherapy—Cold baths and showers are excellent remedies for tiredness, numbness, and general weakness. Take a towel and dip it in cold water and ice and rub it vigorously all over your body (arms, chest, neck, face, calves, and legs). Treat each part of your body with care and attention before moving on to the next.

Nutrition—To cope with the fatigue that sometimes accompanies a state of illness, I like to drink plenty of fluids and get my protein simultaneously. One drink I have regularly is almond milk, protein powder, cacao, and even bananas. I sometimes experiment with different ingredients, like peanut butter or cinnamon, to get an extra boost of energy.

Meditation—Using meditation is a great way to prepare our bodies for starting the day or retiring from one. It's a place that affords us insight and a passageway (a liminal and subliminal space) between the realities of sleep and waking. It's an opportunity for our minds to settle down or recharge for the world of sleep. Personally, when going to bed at night, I like to rely on a body scan technique, with some deep breathing by inhaling through my nose and exhaling through my mouth. I practice this right before going to bed. It's an opportunity to consciously check out my mind, body, and spirit before sleeping.

Nine Mindful Activities to Relax and Recharge

Stress, nervousness, and anxiety are bad for our health. If we do not quickly and compassionately become aware of pressure, it can build up. A quick decompression only takes five minutes. The Nine Mindful Activities below can be used for that purpose. They take five minutes each and will help you "move a muscle and change a thought."

1. Walking

Whether it's in the park or a quiet place, this will immediately relax you. The change will help you deal with stress, and if you are in an office or anywhere, you can take advantage of lunchtime to walk to a nice place somewhere nearby.

It doesn't take long to connect with nature. You only need five minutes to listen to the birds chirping, smell the flowers, look at the sky, and take in the beauty of the world. You can even reflect on something in your head for a moment.

2. Breathing

We always breathe, but we don't always do it consciously. Paying attention to the air that enters your lungs is an excellent idea—breathing is not just a mechanical process. When you become very focused on your breath as a vital life force nourishing your body, it reduces stress levels and allows you to receive even more oxygen.

So, even taking a series of deep breaths (always through your nose) helps you be conscious of the inhalation and exhalation. You don't have to go to a park or the countryside. You can calm down at the office. Close your eyes and put yourself in a comfortable position, sitting, standing, or lying down—it makes no difference.

A helpful exercise is to plug the right nostril and inhale only with the left. Then change and do the same thing with the other. Alternate nostril breathing helps you balance your breath and purify the energy in your body. It also reduces stress levels and helps reduce acid reflux.

3. Visualizing

Daydream or imagine life as it could be, and then live it. Close your eyes and imagine that you are on a Caribbean island while sipping coconut juice or walking on a sandy beach with clear waters and cleansing waves. Or perhaps you are in the countryside with trees and flowers. Imagine an activity and location you like that gives you serenity.

You can take advantage of an ideal future scenario that allows you to reduce your stress levels and broaden your awareness.

The key to this exercise is to know that what you visualize may become your reality and may require more work than you will put into it!

4. Eating

An empty stomach can increase stress and nervousness. If you eat a healthy meal, you will feel satisfied and happy. The positive connections between what happens in your gut and what you perceive in your brain are indisputable.

Eat peacefully, focusing on and enjoying every bite. Mindfully choose healthy foods like an apple, a cereal bar, or dark chocolate, and avoid fatty or high-sugar foods.

5. Plants and flowers

Plants help calm nervousness, offering pure air so you can breathe better. Breathing on plants helps them to grow stronger; they exchange CO_2 for the oxygen we use.

Dedicate yourself to watering your plants, weeding, and even talking to them, as all living things need encouragement. I often notice my blood pressure decreasing and any nervousness disappearing when I garden.

6. Unplugging

Being connected online with your smartphone or computer can increase stress and nervousness. Researchers have found an imbalance in the brain chemistry of people addicted to smartphones and the internet. According to a recent Pew Research Center study, 46 percent of Americans say they could not live without their smartphones.[19] While this is hyperbole, more and more people increasingly depend on their computers, smartphones, and other portable electronic devices for news, information, games, and even the occasional phone call. I have to unplug consciously, and even then, I have a hard time detaching.

This dependence results in sleep loss, insomnia, depression, sleep problems, nightmares, headaches, muscle aches, and red eyes. You need to rest as much as possible for five minutes every two hours, from whatever you are doing. When you get home, be conscious of not spending your time in front of a screen (TV included). Let go of all screen use for at least an hour before going to sleep. Turn off your devices if they are in the room where you sleep.

7. Connecting with nature

Go outside and get a little sun. I go for a walk on the beach, or by the bay, around a park, or near a pond. Smell a rose, see the reflections in the water, and watch people go by, living their lives. When I was living in New York City, I would find some green patch of grass, a tree, or a bush in the park. I also practiced bringing plants to my office and focused on keeping them alive.

8. Having a massage

While it is unnecessary to get a massage every day—although that would be nice—it is beautiful to take care of your body every day with concern, respect, and kindness. With the day's stresses, the mind can signal the body to contract, withdraw, tighten, and tense.

---

19   https://www.pewresearch.org/internet/2015/04/01/
chapter-two-usage-and-attitudes-toward-smartphones/

With your other thumb and index finger, you can exert light pressure on the flesh of your hand between your index and the middle fingers to release tension. The place is between your knuckle and the space between your fingers. You can also do a thumb massage to relax your shoulder and neck.

When you get a headache, there is nothing better than making circular movements on your temples with your eyes closed or rubbing the upper bridge of your nose to let go of the tension between your eyes.

9. Relaxing to music

Some types of music have a tranquilizing effect on your mind. Instrumental, classical, or mantra music is best, as they all have a calming effect on your nervous system and regulate it. There are many types of music or environmental sounds for going to sleep.

Mindful Tips

Finding time to relax is the same as finding time to live better.

Recharging, sleeping, refreshing, and relaxing are your most effective weapons against stress. It is essential to find at least a few minutes to devote to true and healthy peace every day. Don't ignore your need to recharge—it is necessary. Otherwise, the repercussions can compound and have a severe impact on your life.

A succession of hectic days without a moment's pause leads to an increase in stress. Increased stress means having less concentration and energy and being more prone to a foul mood, not counting the damage that excessive stress brings to your health. Try to find the time to experiment with a relaxation activity that suits you best. You can build small oases of peace during the most challenging days by using mindfulness meditation. If you still wonder how you will find the time to practice without losing your mind, it's time to let go and just start.

How do you rate yourself?

Recharge: Sleep and Refresh: Getting enough rest, relaxation, and sleep to feel energized during the day.

How do you rate yourself on a scale of 1 (low) to 5 (high)?

Where are you?

1	2	3	4	5

Where do you want to be?

1	2	3	4	5

Why did you choose this number?

_____

_____

_____

What changes could you make to help you get there?

_____

_____

_____

Source: Personal Health Inventory –
Veterans Affairs. https://www.va.gov/WHOLEHEALTH/docs/10-773_PHI_May2020.pdf

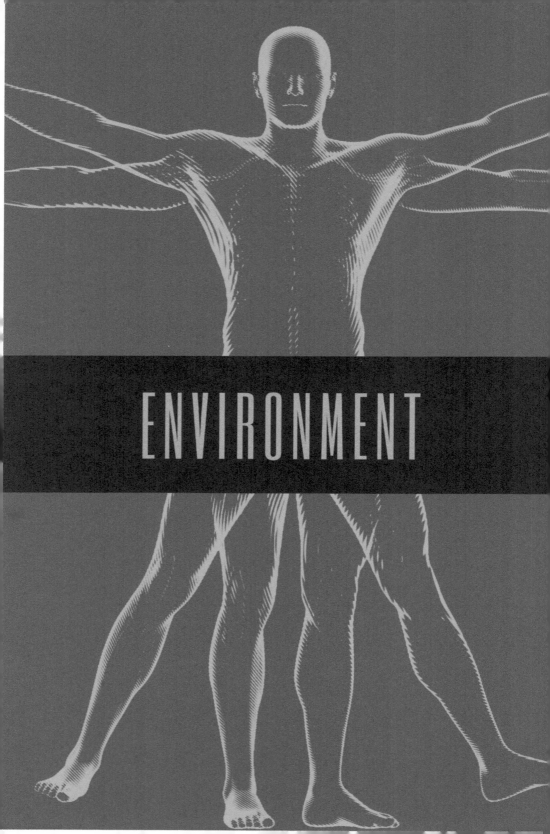

ENVIRONMENT

Chapter 6

ENVIRONMENT

Physical and Emotional

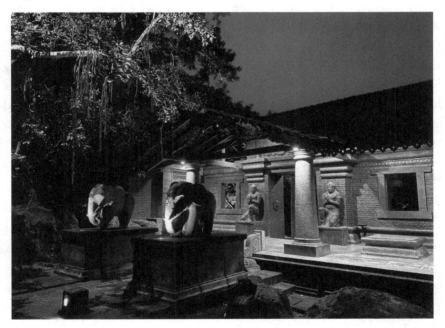

Sense of the sacred,, Elephant Corridor, Entrance to Hotel, Sri Lanka, 2019

WE MOVE FROM looking at mindfulness as a strictly inside job to see how we can create mindful environments. As you work mindfully on yourself, you can bring mindfulness to your daily life to impact the world around you and make visible the kindness and compassion you cultivate. You can reach out and touch your environment and surroundings with loving-kindness and start realizing how you appreciate it. You can create mindful spaces in your home to retreat to, reflect in, and renew yourself. In this part of your mindfulness journey, you can explore all the incredible options you have to create memorable, beautiful, sacred places and spaces to bump your senses and awareness to the next level.

Globally, the pandemic has increasingly made the world a more frantic and stressful place. People are rushing around in survival mode, figuring out health, family, and work commitments. Conserving your energies and cultivating positive energy are essential. Consider your surroundings to find quiet and welcoming spaces that recharge, regenerate, and help you regain strength so you can face your days of frenzy.

Many spaces reflecting current lifestyles are crowded with furniture, accessories, and additional items purchased over time, carrying no meaning or utility. Our rooms might be full of too much stuff. When our homes are overstuffed, they create a chaotic and suffocating effect on our psyches, a feeling of being weighed down, along with an inability to breathe fresh oxygen. We can get lost in the clutter, quite literally. Our minds can become stagnant and crowded with worries and regrets about the past or anxieties about the future. We must stop and get clear, calm, and connected to the present. By surrounding ourselves with an atmosphere that is clear, calm, and connected, we can clear away the chaos of life.

I believe that our work environments and homes store both positive and negative energies. We can intentionally create an atmosphere that matches our outsides to our insides. We can create an environment that helps us change, relax, and inspire the best that we can be. Let's take a deeper dive into this idea of balancing our lives by using our surroundings.

I believe that highly empathic individuals can sense the "emotional residue" that's left in places by people who have experienced happiness, joy, serenity, pain, anger, anxiety, or fear. For the skeptical, the argument is that energy is fluid and gets transferred to walls, floors, and furnishings throughout the surroundings. While not visible to the naked eye, these invisible energies, like transparent varnish, live in the surroundings like lived experiences.

Think of energy in a similar way to radioactive waves that our bodies can feel as helpful, threatening, or neutral. You don't know why you like or don't like a person, place, or thing, but you have an automatic aversion or attraction. These feelings may be due to what is called "harmonic resonance" or the "frequency" of the resident energy field of the human body, which has been tested to resonate at 5 Hz. Human beings are energetic bodies that naturally match each other and the outside world. With mindful awareness, this interconnectedness can help us adjust our environments to either enhance or shield ourselves from the world.

If you've ever walked into a place and felt positive or negative emotions, you understand how energy can impact you. The negative emotions are more solemn, lower, and denser than a vibratory field (think waves and ocean). The positive energy and emotions resonate at a higher vibration and are more energetic and alive. Cluttered spaces are not clean or in tune with the environment. You can fill them with various natural elements to harmonize with spirit, soul, ancestry, aspiration, or divine intelligence.

Ideally, you want to clear your surroundings of toxins, clutter, and bad emotional energies. Clearing out the negative things in your life might involve acceptance, throwing stuff out, and a change of attitude. You might need to excavate old wounds, memories, thoughts, and ideas that no longer serve you. You might need to take the paint off of old furniture and restore it to its natural beauty.

Restoration is about brining your sense of love and compassion back to your life. It might require you to take time off, let go, change, or muster the courage to let go the dreams that didn't work out. The process might involve heat, sound, wind, lighting candles, burning incense (sage to clear the energies in a space), going to old photos, books, or memories.

You need to open the space around you, in your mind, body, and spirit—anything that can help you let go of the old and make way for the new is essential.

Open Up to Serenity Meditation

This meditation is potent. It will open your heart and mind to serenity and affirm your place in the world. It does not matter if you have a large or small space since it involves affirmation, imagination, and visualization. The visualization exercise helps you to envision and imagine wide-open spaces and brightly lit surroundings. You will repeat words like *serenity*, *play*, and *peace*. Write these words down on paper or your phone and hold them in your hand.

Now, sit and focus on the words with your eyes closed and think of a time in your life when you had space and when you were serene or felt peaceful. Where were you? What were you doing? Think of one time or a collection of memories. What was happening? Were you on a beach, a mountain, at a retreat center, or in a forest? What elements were present in your visualization, water, fire, air, trees, rocks?

Open your eyes and bring these elements and the idea of this serene space to your interior surroundings. Focus on individual spaces, corners, and places in each of your rooms. Bring these ideas to where you work, where you play, and where you sleep. How do you bring light and color to empty spaces and textures? Where is nature and ritual, and where are your ancestors?

Look to create more spaces in various rooms and areas. Do it with all the drama and emotion a movie set designer might use. You want to create spaces for yourself and other people to enjoy. Treat the people who come into your environment with areas that are alive and have meaning, a story, and a sense of energy that helps them thrive.

Calming your nervous system

You can go beyond the basics of safety and security by focusing on physical comfort, temperature, air quality, and the physical elements that help you be psychologically comfortable, relaxed, and at ease. I love using external stimuli to evoke insight and heightened awareness in my interior world. I incorporate lighting, sound, and texture to influence perception, emotion, and my thoughts with color, sound, texture, smell, light, shadow, highlights, artwork arrangements, decor, and furniture. With the proper staging of your environment, you can enhance concepts with visual elements that flow into your everyday living, working, and enjoyment of life.

Colors

If you're not sure how to do this, start with colors, hues, and lighting to impact your mood or cognitive function. Look into the practice of color psychology—the study of shades of color as a determinant of human behavior. Color influences perceptions, such as the taste of food, and color can cause specific emotions in people. Shades of red and orange stand for passion and help boost energy. Shades of gray and blue promote tranquility and relaxation and are suitable for high-traffic areas, such as the kitchen and living room. White is a classic color that exudes purity and calmness, making it ideal for small or poorly lit spaces. Yellow and green symbolize creativity, prosperity, and natural sparkle, whereas black and purple connote royalty and power.

How you use the colors in primary or secondary combinations is essential. Using lighting and ambient colors allows you to spotlight specific areas or bring out the depths of shade resonant in objects. There are several light kits that you can use to highlight the environment. I like Phillips Hue lighting kits, which offer many options for configuring a space, whether it's a home, office, or retail location.

Tell your story

Your surroundings should be an extension and expression of your story, aspirations, intentions, and personality. Your work environment is the same, as you want to physically illustrate your branding, vision, and values that you wish to bring into the world. Select elements that allow this to take shape with photos, water, candles, flowers, plants, murals, icons, and statues. These things can be emotionally and aesthetically pleasing. Yet aesthetics can also be practical—flowers, plants, or trees provide oxygen and moisture to the environment. Creating mindful surroundings is an art form that has been around for centuries. It's the art of Feng Shui.

Feng Shui

Pronounced *fung shway*, this term means "wind and water." Its roots are 5,000 years old. Feng shui seeks to promote prosperity, exceptional health, and general well-being by examining how energy, *qi* (pronounced *chee*), flows through a particular room, house, building, or garden. You can learn a lot from this ancient art of energetic placement to furnish your surroundings harmoniously. As a guideline, choose materials, objects, and color placement that help you create an atmosphere of peace and harmony following nature's flow. According to Chinese tradition, the order of furniture and natural elements helps amplify health, wellness, and happiness by promoting open space, allowing your life-force energies to flow and be in better harmony with your environment.

According to feng shui, clutter blocks the natural flow of energy and has no place in a well-designed interior. Being diligent and vigilant in this practice requires that you throw away broken or useless items and let go of the things you no longer need. Bring life and color into your living or workspaces to brighten them up and attract prosperity, positive vibes, and focus.

Feng shui offers guidance to harmonize space and to draw energy and benefits from the surroundings. Many people have entered a home or office and felt relaxed, confused, or tired and weighed down by the environment. Feng shui focuses on creating places that feel agreeable, so you get a complete sense of well-being in them. You can take care of dark areas that don't feel right with lights, plants, colors, or elements of nature that help to lighten and brighten the surroundings.

Based on your date, time, and place of birth, feng shui focuses on a person's energies to determine the most suitable locations for placing objects, the elements. Some elements have a cyclic nature, with yin, receptive energy, and yang, active energy. These energies are ever engaged in a dance, seeking power, flow, harmony, and balance in nature. When empowered, we are "harmonized" in our relationships with others. The purpose of feng shui is to bring peace to ourselves and our environment.

Feng Shui Remedies

By rebalancing energies, you strive to use plants, mirrors, lights, or colors to design surroundings and enhance and brighten the space. We should never place plants in a bedroom because energetically, they can disturb sound sleep. They are ideal in the bathroom, helping to rebalance the room's predominant element (water). Mirrors are also important because they can reflect energy but are "off-putting" in an entrance. Mirrors are ideal for tight spaces because they expand a long and narrow corridor or a too-small room.

The use of light, according to the rules of feng shui, is crucial. Rooms with yang (powerful) energies, dedicated to activities like cooking or study, should be well lit. Delicate, sweeter energy rooms are more yin (receptive) and are devoted to rest and spirituality, such as the bedroom or living room. Yin energy is more indirect, so lighting is subdued or moody. With the use of both yin and yang energies, the use of color is significant. For example, red is out of place in the house's yin rooms and the bathroom, contrasting with the predominant water element (blue). Yellow is ideal in the kitchen, green in the children's room and the bathroom, and light blue in the bedroom. Lighter colors and accents are always up to personal taste.

Creating the world around you is like painting or photographing a collage for your life's memories. It can be a lot of fun. You don't need to be concerned or worried if you are doing it right. You can use various elements and colors in rooms and experiment to see if the changes in lighting or arrangement impact your perception of the space, change your energy, or lift and shift your mood.

It's suitable for your outward life to reflect your inner values, intentions, and personal brand. You can exemplify your energies with the placement of color, light, and space. If you neglect your surroundings or your area has negative energy, you will feel it. This negative energy is inside and outside of your body and your environment. It's a beneficial idea to ensure that your "inner house" reflects authentically to the world outside. People spread their energies to other people, places, and things just by being present. Sweetness or stink have their smells.

The principles of harmony and prosperity in feng shui are thousands of years old and still lived within the walls of your home, office, or surroundings. When you create mindful spaces, it enables you to be relaxed, creative, and focused on making yourself and others happy and productive.

Here are ten ideas inspired by feng shui's principles to create a happy, healthy, and welcoming environment and improve the appearance and energies of your spaces. They will enhance each room's appearance to accommodate all the points linked to life, work, and success. I believe that there is no better investment of time in life than reorganizing and decorating your home or office to make your life more beautiful, breathable, and livable. So, give this your full attention and put your mind, body, and spirit into this activity.

1. Entrance

The entrance is a symbol of prosperity and hospitality. So, your front door, as well as the surrounding area, should always be in perfect condition. Place a wreath or planter near the door and position a lush green plant (a welcome greeter) nearby to attract positive energy into the entrance. Don't forget the proper lighting will highlight the area and stress the perception of depth. Through this doorway, you enter your world of intimate relationships, emotions, soul, and spirit. The entrance represents a portal into a more vulnerable part of life, separated from the outside world. You step through the doorway into a sacred place of dreams and possibilities.

2. Hallways

Hallways are the "main streets" of your home or office. You need to keep them clean and orderly, just as you would an airport runway for flight take-off or landing. Keep the hallway free from any obstacle, garbage, or clutter, to allow energy to circulate, letting people move in, out, and about. Use closets to store clothes and shoes. If you can, keep a mirror, candles, flowers, and a bit of greenery to fill the space with positivity, light, and energy. Your entrance and departure points provide the transition from one way of being to another. You move from the world outside to the sanctuary of your home or workplace. Make these changes mindfully and with intention.

3. Living/Meeting Rooms

Relaxation, collaboration, sharing, and creation happen here. It's where excellence has the space to flourish. The room should be large enough for all gatherings and orderly with furniture and lighting that does not overwhelm (bright white lights), yet supports comfort and utility. Leave the doors open and free from obstacles, and position furniture against or near a wall to help those wishing to sit and gather. Again, use lighting to enhance the energy and harmony of the room. Use lamps (soft lighting) in the corners diagonally opposite the entrance door to accent plants, artwork, or mood.

4. Kitchen

Kitchens are our actual living spaces. They are where you get food, nourishment, and harmony. You don't need the kitchen to be loud, so tone down the colors, and avoid bright oranges, reds or black, and dark brown shades. You don't want your kitchen to be reminiscent of incidents with flames, water, or waste. If you are designing your kitchen, it's best not to place the sink and stove next to each other, as water and fire don't mix. Keep the garbage near the sink for cleaning and disposing of waste.

5. Dining room

Like the kitchen, your dining room is vital for feng shui because it represents the sharing of food as a source of energy, life, and sustenance. Keep the dining room happy with fresh flowers, candles that optimize the space's power, and lights to accent its mood. Put a mirror on the wall to reflect the table's sacred ambiance with its candles, where you will enjoy a meal together.

6. Bedroom

While chapter 5 is all about recharging and sleep, it's crucial to outline that the bedroom needs to have the right feng shui. You don't want the bedroom in an area with a lot of traffic, so do your best to make it the most secluded area of your house, and use neutral colors to promote restful sleep. The position of the bed is also essential. The headboard always goes against a wall and, if possible, not in line with the door. For balance and symmetry, place two identical nightstands on each side of the bed and place soft light lamps and a few candles to create a relaxed atmosphere. It's best not to bring the television into the bedroom, as you want to make this the place where you let go of the outside world and nurture your inside world mindfully, with rest and sleep.

7. Children's room

Like your bedroom, you want to ensure the children's room is secluded too. If possible, face the headboard southeast/southwest to increase creativity and offer your child the best sleep. Use light and pastel shades, natural wood floors, and wall lighting for the entire room. Essential lights near the bed, and an indirect night-light, are acceptable as needed. Use music boxes and pinwheels hanging from the ceiling. Checkered fabric decorations also generate a balancing effect and recall vital energy.

8. Offices

The office is the money area, and you want to position your desk where you always have control over everything that happens around it. The desk should face the door and be angled in such a way that you feel like you are in control of the space Do your best to have it neat and uncluttered so that positive news is welcome. I like to have landscape paintings, family photographs, and plants to create a relaxed atmosphere. Pay attention to electrical appliances, outlets, and access for meetings and communication. Ease of access is essential for network connections.

9. Bathroom

The bathroom is essential for all of us from cleanliness and security viewpoints. Figuratively and literally, it's the place where you wash away the waste and dirt of your life. Keeping it clean, with doors that close and a toilet lid that lowers is essential. Figuratively, water drains wealth, so it is better to include some plants nearby, which will slow the flow of wealth and energy as the water goes down the drain.

10. Garden

If you are lucky enough to be out of a crowded city, this is one of the most critical aspects of your environment to me. Keeping a garden near the house or office allows you to connect with your essential nature and get in touch with caring for something more than yourself. Even if you are in a city, it does not matter how big it is. Putting it on a veranda, terrace, or just finding a small green space inside is fine. The key is to be mindful and future-oriented for the energetic aspects needed to keep your garden alive and in vigorous condition. Plants, flowers, spices, vegetables, etc., require wholesome soil and attention to feeding, weeding, and growing. You might want to place plants throughout your space to invigorate, revitalize, and encourage your commitment to life and prosperity. Just be mindful about keeping them alive and well-watered!

Sacred spaces

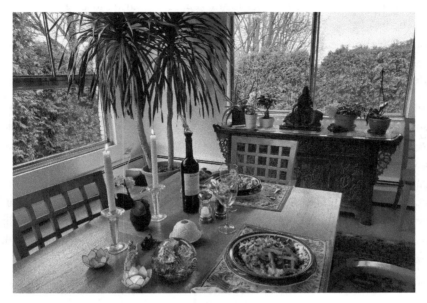

Vegan dinner, candlelight, music, lights, 2020

Sacred spaces are places where you can relax, meditate, and recharge your energies. Your life needs to be surrounded by whatever is sacred to you. These are not religious places—although they can be—yet they offer opportunities for you to reflect and recharge your spirit as a human being, not a "human doing."

You put the world behind yourself and enter a liminal space, a transitional or transformative space, the waiting area between one point in time and space and the next. Often, when you are in a liminal space, you feel that you are in between but on the verge of something. In these spaces, you pay homage to your inside and invite yourself to be even more on the inside. You allow yourself to reach deep inside for inner peace and authentic awareness of yourself and the surrounding world. I invite you now to find the right place—a small corner or center space—to be in the here and now.

The first step is to find the right place in your home or office, a place that may be discreet or in the corner of a living area, meeting space, or meditation room. Remember that you can always ask an expert to help find the right place and balance it with your décor.

Colors are a fundamental and essential part of your meditation oasis. Select natural and warm colors for your liminal space; let nature inspire the area. All the shades of sand and earth with green vegetation or blue-water accents create tranquility and peace for your senses and mind.

Music

Your mind produces brain wave patterns strongly influenced by music. Music activates specific neural circuits, affects cognitive development, and is an essential "lubricant" for the creative process. Many neurological studies have documented the importance of music for the mind. Robert Zatorre, a Canadian neurologist, discovered that music lights up our brains' dopamine-receptor pleasure centers.[20] Like eating or sex, music fires the areas of pleasure and connection. We are wired for music, physically and spiritually. Music has played a role in primitive societies, accompanies rituals, and connects us to the universe's song and sound.

Studies show that the right music can help us calm down, to be in the flow, move us to tears, or make us dance. Music (like all activities related to emotions and art) activates our brains' right hemisphere, responsible for spatial tasks, musical and artistic endeavors, body control, awareness, creativity, and imagination. Consider music as a universal language, experienced by all, which helps us develop conscious experiences at home, in the car, or office.

In my house, I try different types of music and sounds at various times of the day or evening to evoke experiences or moods that strike the occasion. Try out a few ambient sounds (the sound of a fire, a waterfall, or a rainstorm), jazz, electronic beats, rock, or heavy metal (think motorcycle shop). If you want to chill, try Tibetan bowls, Om sound vibrations, or sounds of nature. The more you experiment with your surroundings, the more likely you will create more pleasant and relaxing spaces for both your body and mind.

---

20   https://www.psypost.org/2019/02/
listening-to-the-music-you-love-will-make-your-brain-release-more-dopamine-study-finds-53059

Minimal and natural furnishings

I like spaces that are free of clutter. I want to have a few furnishings and accessories that are simple, with fine lines and open spaces. I like aspirational areas, evoking a sense of peace and order. Like wood, bamboo, wicker, and paper—natural materials seem to work best and produce grounding and calm.

Relaxing light

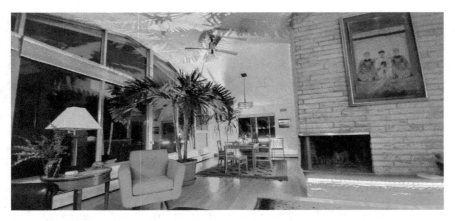

Lights, plants, water, candles and music enriches our environment, 2020

I like the use of natural light for meditation. But a large window or a skylight is even better. Use glowing lights or candles to spread a warm glow for a sacred atmosphere. Set the intention for your space, noting the shadows and tones, but keeping the area bathed in soft, warm lighting.

Adding a bit of green

Adding a fern or a bonsai for the green in your Zen corner is a beautiful addition. Just be sure to water per the instructions, as these can be challenging to keep. You could also use clippings and put them in a simple, small jar. Greenery encourages meditation and instills peace and tranquility by recalling nature in your meditation corner.

Water

I've incorporated water bowls in our meditation corner because water is a beneficial element. You might find a small indoor fountain with a delicate sound to help soothe stress, promote relaxation, and create a positive energy flow. But even simple water bowls can help you to balance energy in a room. They come in all types and sizes, from the simplest to the most complex, some with various light or color effects.

Zen garden

A Zen garden is an open space organized according to the principles of feng shui. You can have a small-scale garden by placing a bonsai onto a simple wooden tray and positioning it where you prefer.

Every element in a Zen garden has a deep and precise meaning as well as an aesthetic function. A Zen garden in Japanese culture is minimalist and, in most cases, a dry garden. You can find its three elements in large open spaces and mini-Zen gardens.

- **Water** symbolizes life and the passing of time and is represented by sand or gravel. There may be small waterfalls, fountains, or ponds outside or indoor Zen fountains for enclosed spaces.

- **Rocks** represent nature and the mountains, and they are a symbol of solidity and peace. Stones are never of the same color or same form and celebrate the soul's steadfast spirit and irregularity.

- **Vegetation** is not always present, especially in indoor Zen gardens. If you want to make vegetation part of your cozy corner, ferns and moss are generally used, not many flowering plants (rhododendron, camellia, or azalea).

Mini-Zen gardens that you can keep at home or on your desk bring this philosophy inside. It's something to do when you are just sitting, and your mind wanders. Take care of it by gently raking the sand and symbolically creating waves like a sea. It will help you create an open meditation that calls you to let go of the clutter and be at peace.

Aromatherapy

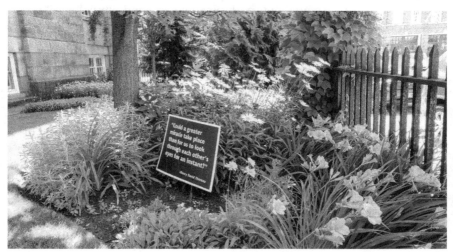

The intoxicating smell of flowers in a churchyard in Portsmouth, NH, 2019

Aromatherapy is another way to brighten and lighten your atmosphere and yourself. Essential oils are natural remedies extracted from the leaves, flowers, and barks of plants. The extraction method enables the oil to maintain its medicinal properties that lend themselves to different uses. Thus, it is always helpful to have oils at home for cleaning or the atmosphere.

I use many and varied essential oils in aromatherapy. Each has specific properties that, once known, can be exploited for different needs. There is no need to have an extensive collection of them, though I find it difficult to resist the temptation to experiment with new ones. Different oils impact your mind, body, spirit, and emotions in particular ways. So, I like to see how I feel after applying them and whether I feel any different.

Essential oils smell fabulous. I like to use them in a diffuser with water or apply them to my skin. They are best mixed with raw vegetable oil (such as sweet almond oil or sesame oil) or with cream, should you wish to spread the smell on your skin. It requires only a tiny number of drops to achieve the desired effect. Essential oils are fifty times more potent than the plants or herbs they come from. They can have strong antibacterial properties, fight germs, and prevent infections. Their aroma acts on our limbic system, connected to areas of our brains that control heart rate, blood pressure, breathing, stress levels, and memory. With essential oils, both psychological and physiological effects occur in the mind and body.

For example, think of the relaxing properties of lavender essential oil. If you use it on the burner or sprinkle a few drops on a handkerchief to smell it, you realize that your mind and body relax little by little. Lavender is best used for relaxing when you find it hard to sleep. Recent scientific studies have shown that rosemary essential oil can improve memory precisely because of its fragrance. Would that help you with your work or personal life?

Essential oils help our bodies heal because they strengthen the immune system and act against bacteria that cause problems and diseases. Essential oils help the body regain its natural balance.

Although they are natural remedies, we must use essential oils with caution, always under the guidance of an herbalist, a pharmacist, or an expert. Using essential oils with children under the age of three has contraindications. Pregnant or lactating women might have an allergic reaction to an herbal mix or its strength. Careless application of pure essential oils on the skin can cause injury.

It's always appropriate to dilute them in oil or cream and follow an expert's advice. The contraindications depend on the dose and how the essential oils are used with your health conditions or problems. For this reason, when it comes to choosing essential oils as a curative remedy, it's wise to turn to a trusted expert.

Application and use of essential oils

Here are some ideas on where you might use essential oils in your house.

- **At the entrance**

  Essential oils extracted from citrus fruits (lemon, orange, cedar, bergamot, grapefruit) have an energizing effect. They give you a boost of vitality to face the day and welcome you with a vibrant note when you return home tired.

- **In the bathroom**

  Lavender has a natural relaxing effect, which induces sleep by calming the body and mind. You can put a few drops directly into the tub and inhale the vapors while you enjoy a hot bath before going to bed. The psychophysical benefits are instantaneous!

- **In the kitchen**

  If a cooking odor remains even after changing the air, the essential oils of mint, Scotch pine, and eucalyptus purify the air, leaving it pleasantly balsamic. They also stimulate concentration if your children are doing their homework.

- **In the living room**

  If you like a classic clean scent, focus on the essential oil of ylang-ylang. If you want fragrant air, such as a spring mix of woody and floral essences, use sandalwood, flowers, and vanilla to give an exotic touch.

- **In the study**

  If you work at home, bitter orange gives you determination and focus. Jasmine gives you a sense of well-being and optimism to meet your commitments with positivity.

- **In the bedroom**

  To keep away a cold or the flu and clear the airways while you sleep, use thyme, which has a mild antibacterial effect. To awaken the passions, choose patchouli for its aphrodisiac properties.

- **In the children's bedroom**

  To wish your children sweet dreams put a few drops of blue chamomile in a bowl on the bedside table. It is one of the safest and most recommended essential oils for children.

I like to think of using essential oils in combination with water, bathing, or grooming. It's a perfect way to nourish the skin and bathe your body with kindness. Make sure to focus and concentrate, with loving-kindness, to super-charge their impact and effect as you apply them.

Mindful Tips

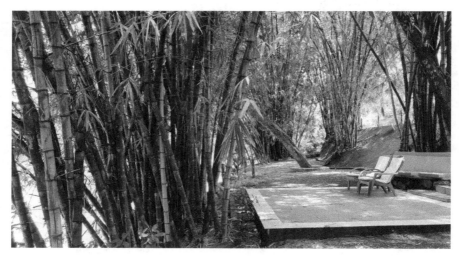

Relaxation Space, Mekosha Ayurvedic Retreat Center, Kerala, India, 2019

In summary, I believe that life is a significant ritual—that everything you do can involve patterns—and how you pay attention to your surroundings is an essential step in making your life divine.

In his book, *The Miracle Morning*, Hal Elrod identifies the combination of six steps to create a ritual that can help you live the life you want. They are essential for creating a morning miracle that gives you as much as you invest in your self-care.

- **Silence**: Closing your eyes and focusing on your breathing is more than enough to start eliminating stress.

- **Affirmation**: Defining and doing what you want in your life is the first step to change.

- **Visualization**: Because words become deeds, it is necessary to imagine them first. What is a visual representation of your life? What do you see in your mind's eye and believe you can manifest and achieve in the physical world? To induce change, believe in it and behave as if that change has already happened. It's like a flight simulator. You imagine what things would be like, and this helps you take the path forward toward action.

- **Physical exercise**: This prepares your body for the day.

- **Reading**: This is to learn something new every day.

- **Writing**: This is a means of meditation and analysis to focus on personal growth and define your purpose, meaning, and gratitude.

Create an energetic environment

What is the secret to being reinvigorated in an instant? Make the natural light reflect. Play with it. Use mirrors, other materials, or bright colors to reflect it. Your interior will be more radiant, and you will feel full of energy!

Green plants!

Plants have a calming effect. They supply oxygen, and the green color transmits calm and serenity.

Clean and tidy

Order and cleanliness are essential to ensure that the flow of energy can circulate.

Colors and lights

Play with colors and lights to reduce stress and create a calm environment. Creating mindful surroundings is an incredible way to shift your perspective, live in the present moment, and have places you can call your own where you chill out, let your defenses down, and live in a healthier, happier way.

How do you rate yourself?

Environment: *Physical and Emotional*

Having comfortable, healthy spaces where you work and live—the quality of the lighting, color, air, and water: decreasing unpleasant clutter, noises, and smells.

How do you rate yourself on a scale of 1 (low) to 5 (high)?

Where are you?

1	2	3	4	5

Where do you want to be?

1	2	3	4	5

Why did you choose this number?

What changes could you make to help you get there?

Source: Personal Health Inventory –

Veterans Affairs. https://www.va.gov/WHOLEHEALTH/docs/10-773_PHI_May2020.pdf

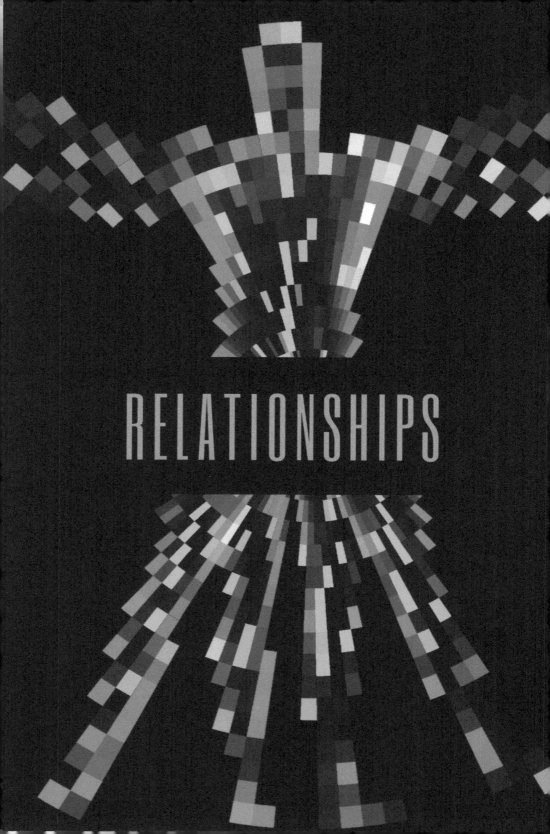

RELATIONSHIPS

Chapter 7

RELATIONSHIPS

Love, Friends, and Marriage

THIS CHAPTER EXPLORES how we can be more mindful in our relationships with others. It offers perspectives on healthy boundaries in your relationships and ways of communicating to create conscious, safe spaces where you can live in a relationship.

During my lifetime, I have found that feeling alone sometimes makes me sick or keeps me sick. It's almost as if I feel like I have lost a part of myself. It's the hole in the soul that longs for the connection to be whole.

We human beings are wired and programmed for connection. We are in relationships with others. When we have positive social relationships, we just feel healthy. A healthy mind, body, and intimate relationship with a partner can be a source of strength. My most tremendous achievement in life is having failed in relationships at an early age. That failure helped me investigate myself further and try harder to develop ties to people I could talk to, who equally cared about our stories, journeys, and concerns.

Our early childhood attachments form the basis for our relationship with the world. Through them, we feel secure with who we are and our place in the world. We can also feel insecure or scattered by them, given the time and attention invested in the relationship. Feeling alone can be a dark place where negativities develop. You can think that you are alone, feel lonely, and ill at ease with life, friends, and family during those periods. It is best to distance yourself from people, places, and things that do not feed your soul or support you, or even worse, hurt you. When this happens, I like to say, "I wish you well, even love and happiness, but far, far away from me." To have a healthy perspective, you need to cultivate kindhearted relationships with friends, family, and co-workers. You need to be safe and contain your relations to navigate life toward a chosen destination, secure in knowing that you are safe, and live life to the fullest!

Positive Relationships

Positive relationships are healthy. A healthy, intimate relationship with a life partner can be a source of strength. It's wise to talk with people who care about you and listen. To be happy in life, we need to cultivate relationships with others! When we do, we feel seen, heard, recognized, and validated. It is one secret to having a happy and satisfying life.

Lives are like gardens. Human beings and gardens both live by breathing, needing nourishment to grow and develop—fertilizer and manure to grow seeds of love, compassion, and conscious intention to weed and water, providing bright light for flourishing.

Many studies conducted in social psychology have shown that those with a satisfying emotional and relational life are much happier, have better health, and live longer. When it is not a voluntary choice, being alone can harm our psychological well-being more than we can imagine, leading to a sense of worthlessness.

The feeling of worthlessness, not being necessary to anyone, causes individuals to sink into depression and even suicide. This kind of loneliness is spreading more and more, aided by the frenetic rhythms of contemporary life and, more recently, COVID, which has impacted millions of lives worldwide. People have lost their jobs, homes, and connections to their community. When they drop out and fall into the network feed of introverted synthetic relationships, they are more connected to the increasingly digital, dystopian world of media, news, reality television, movies, pop culture, and extroversion. Real physical connections, which are emotionally supportive, become even more critical as they fulfill the deep need for meaningful human contact.

Lonely people may be shy, have poor social skills, distrust others, or not be emotionally intelligent or socialized. Loneliness can be defeated by attempting to get out of one's shell and open to others through writing, art, nature, and group mashups. There are online communities to join.

The most significant relationship we can ever have is with ourselves. This one relationship will last a lifetime, and it requires us to be still and open to whatever arises and trust our instincts. Everyone is different, but we are alike in so many ways. We all express happiness and sadness the same way. We all feel moved, touched, and inspired by something or someone. For some of us, though, some of those feelings were traumatized or damaged.

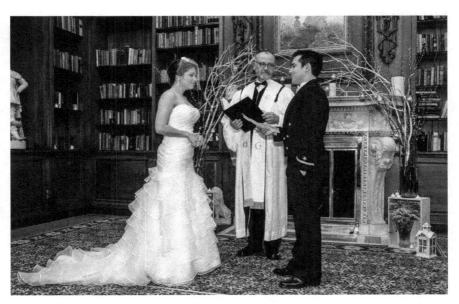

Wedding ceremony of my nephew and his bride, 2014

Attempt to make new friends

After high school or college, it becomes more challenging to make new friends. We have less time, and we get busy with work and family. Everyone has their life, and there is less willingness to meet new people or venture off. Even with old friends, it may not feel the same as it was in the past. Many things change from adolescence to adulthood, and our old friends may have taken a completely different direction than us.

If you want new friendships, you must devote yourself to your social life. It takes time to focus your energies to create opportunities to meet other people. Before the COVID pandemic, you could go to places where people congregate—a gym, a volunteer program, a dance course, or a theater. You could go to concerts, festivals, or make group trips. Choices are much more limited with the pandemic, and much of what you can do now is online. The important thing is to do your best to interact with the people you meet and discuss meaningful or controversial topics. There are multiple places and things you can do to network in these communities. Check out the websites Eventbrite or Meetup or look at your local online newspaper for Zoom activities.

Make the first move

It is easier to make friends if you make social contact. However, taking the first step can be difficult if you are a shy person. To reduce your anxiety, be mindful and remember that all people, even those who seem brilliant and winning, have their fears and insecurities—maybe they feel just as alone as you. So, exercise empathy and compassion.

Many of us fear others will notice our flaws and our darkest secrets and reject us once we get close. But everyone wants to be seen, heard, and recognized. Being shy is often characterized by excessive self-awareness. So, focus on the person in front of you, who may have the same insecurities and issues. You may be surprised to find that what flows through you flows through them. There are opportunities to connect with each other's experiences.

Be who you are

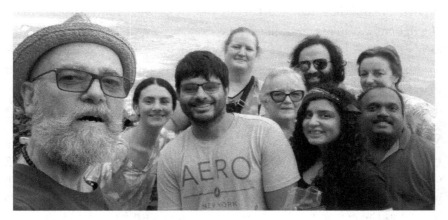

New friends, Ayurvedic Retreat, Kerala, India 2019

When you first meet someone and say hello, what matters is not whether you look exciting or entertaining. It is more important that you are who you are and be as present as possible with the person and situation. Being aware of your breathing and energy and taking an interest in the other person's feelings is one of the keys to cultivating successful friendships.

> *You can make more friends in two months, being interested in others, than in two years trying to make people take an interest in you.*
>
> —DALE CARNEGIE

Intimacy (or Into-Me-See)

It takes time to build trust. Building trust is like creating a sound foundation when you are constructing a home. Oversharing too early, physically or emotionally, before laying down a firm foundation can ruin friendship prospects. It is better to be friendly and social but avoid confidences at the beginning—such as, "Last week I seriously considered suicide." These kinds of confessions can scare or embarrass a new acquaintance. Take the time to know the other person and exchange ideas, feelings, and physical intimacies slowly. I believe that this approach is always suitable.

Be yourself

It doesn't matter how rich and famous you are or what your social life looks like right now. You may be feeling alone, even in a crowd. You may have all the cash and prizes, but you still feel lonely. It can be even worse when you have wealth; you wonder if people are there for you because of what you have rather than who you are.

As Oscar Wilde so brilliantly said, "Be yourself; everyone else is already taken."

When you pretend to be healthier, brighter, and confident while hurting inside, it is challenging to experience real intimacy. If you have a painful feeling of loneliness, you can feel as if no one understands you. You need to stop pretending to be the person who others expect you to be and allow yourself to be seen as the person you are. Take your time in turning acquaintances into friends. You can find strength in vulnerability and develop genuine friendships in good and bad times. Everyone has a judge or critic, and it's often best to shine a light on it to quieten it.

Quiet the critic

Do not size people up too quickly, reject them, or adopt a rigid or critical attitude. When you expect too much in relationships and hold an idealized concept of friendship, you may be quickly disappointed. You may prefer breaking up a friendship rather than taking responsibility for your position and realizing that even confessing your judgments and criticisms might bring the relationship closer. When you compare and despair, you measure others and use offense to support your weak position. You may practice one-upmanship and continually try to win over friends and family because you need to feel superior.

People are socialized differently and reciprocate, acknowledge, understand, and communicate in different ways. By being mindful of others, and yourself, you can be more tolerant and not expect anything from others. The more you can do this, the better you will be in a relationship with others. Everyone has a blind spot. We are all challenged in different ways to show up for life. Acceptance and a more nonjudgmental attitude will win friends and influence others.

Healthy vs. Toxic Relationships

We grow healthy relationships in fertile ground, wrapped in sincerity, trust, hope, and a willingness to let go, be in the flow, and move on. When you or others make power moves with sarcasm, bombastic wit, or insincerity, it can feel like manipulation and lead to disastrous outcomes. Manipulative tactics can be relationship killers. Tone, context, or semantics may be missed, especially when texting, emailing, or using social media.

Check your own and your partner's intentions consistently, and make sure that your views align with how you speak, act, and live in the moment for ongoing validation of ideas, speech, mind, and feelings. Love is an intention, a way of being, and honoring each other even though you may disagree. Sharing is an essential factor in any relationship, and it requires special attention and a willingness to implement a process.

Six key ideas or guidelines for relationships

1. Generosity

We base lasting relationships on the generosity of both partners. You need to forgive and forget and move on. Genuine love requires courage expecting nothing in return. What you feel when you give yourself unconditionally has no comparison. It will be best if you are 100 percent Honest, Open, and Willing (HOW) in it for it to work. Trust and mutual support are essential.

2. Acceptance

When there is mutual acceptance, wisdom can emerge, and you can be more natural. In the beginning, you might not know who the other person is, but you can be sure that there will be challenging issues. Care, patience, and negotiation need to be present in your conversations with each other.

You cannot change other people or trick them into doing what you want them to do. You can tell your partner, friend, or lover, what your needs are, and to the best of their capabilities, they can meet you. Relationships grow when each individual is clear about who they are and hopeful that the other can meet and support them as best as possible.

3. Desire

Communication is the fuel that helps build and keep relationships running. Yet, desire, attraction, and the need to have your way can impede building a relationship. Many people today feel they can find love by swiping left or right, and after having sex, they try to develop a relationship. It's like building a house by starting with the roof rather than a foundation of trust and mutual respect. Communication is the gasoline that powers the engine of any relationship. Without it, your connection will not take you very far.

4. Confidentiality

Relationships require confidentiality, especially when communication reveals vulnerabilities and exposes the weaknesses of your mutual passions, past mistakes, and imperfections. Confidentiality is the litmus test of a relationship. To be in a relationship, you feel that your stories, experiences, hurts, pains, shadows, sensitivities, and weaknesses are honored and entrusted to your partner, friends, and loved ones for safekeeping. When someone empowers you and tells you their story, consider yourself lucky that you've gotten to hear someone else's vulnerabilities, and apply the utmost discretion and care.

A relationship can easily collapse when there is a lack of respect. Sacredness surrounds what hides in the soul of every person, especially in the dark shadows. In a couple's life, secrets and hurtful events are not worth mentioning for the relationship's sake. You don't need to tell them to others. You must hold and reserve a space for exceptional people. Relationships require trust, and you must trust the other person to keep in confidence your most private matters.

5. Understanding

We all have quarrels and not-so-pleasant moments with our friends, partners, or as a couple. There are moments when you want to argue and fight to prove you are right and the other person is wrong. The best relationships thrive and endure after disagreements. But holding and maintaining a kind of "I'm right" attitude does not strengthen your bond with the other. The best thing you can do is move on with an eye for understanding. Understand why the other person reacts or thinks the way they do. If you can do that, you will better understand them and yourself. To the extent of your value system, you can meet them where they are. If what someone does is reprehensible, you need to consider your values and others and decide if it is worth investing time in the relationship to understand their actions better. It is only through your relationships that you can come to understand yourself better.

6. Attunement

When friends become united, there is little that can divide them. Emotional attunement allows each individual to sync with the other and feel that the relationship is a balanced two-way street. What a gift when you can be with someone else who gives back to you and is in tune with your thoughts and feelings! Attunement is conscious when you tune into others, synchronizing with their dreams, desires, and goals. Without losing yourself, you intentionally listen to the other, and the "I" becomes "we" to support the other.

You can practice energetic exercises together to gain further attunement and emotionally coregulate. Try breathing together, eye gazing, mutual mindful listening, and speaking, where one person shares and speaks their truth, and the other listens, without talking, nodding, or giving feedback.

Five-minute sharing practice

This is a robust format for a couple, parent, or child, and it is simple to use. Too often, life swallows the necessary time for truer sharing, the sort that deepens connections, reminds us of our craving for intimacy. A five-minute format opens a window for "into-me-see" and a relationship between a couple or small group. Regular practice deepens the sharing.

How it works

- Each person has five minutes to express what they're feeling, or just overall what life feels like at that moment. In contrast with a factual description of the day's events, a five-minute share focuses on the person's feelings. It is like checking in, but only two who know each other very well take part. They have an intimate relationship already, and the five-minute share allows a deeper dive, going beyond the day's events or stories. It's essential to use "I," not "you," statements and expressions of feelings. That way, you take responsibility for your feelings instead of projecting or blaming others for what you are feeling.

- For example, instead of saying, "You made me feel lousy today," you might say, "I feel lousy today, blue, discouraged." In most conversations, the natural response from the other person is "Why?" However, that is not allowed in this exercise. A five-minute share is sacrosanct and without interruption, no matter what is being shared. In fact, no feedback is permitted at the end either. Why? Because it feels safer when you know you can speak, and no one will react, interrupt, or judge. While that might occur in the other's mind, the person sharing feels secure in the silence.

- Often, once one has shared, the other will say during their five-minute share, "You know I feel the same way." For example, "I miss the physical intimacy we have had in the past. I long for more touch, more time to play as we used to." Because the other person is not expected or allowed to react, no debate or defensiveness derails the share. You are practicing mindful listening and sharing. Your feelings are yours. You and your partner are sharing them without interruption. At the end of the share, "feedback" is only offered if you, or the person you share with, want it. If a couple practices a five-minute share every morning, it becomes pretty natural. Their level of intimacy naturally increases as each feels far more aware of what is going on with the other.

Common Mistakes

In relationships, we need to be seen, heard, touched, socialize, and evolve as human beings. No human being is an island. We are all part of an excellent patchwork design made of the over seven billion people on the planet. We all have an essential role in the quality of our connected existence. Relationships provide us with the recognition to live a well-spent life. Without relationships and mutual signs of recognition, care, and comfort, we could not survive. We would not develop as human beings; we'd die.

The fact is that it is better to have poor relationships than none! Relationships are like a mirror to us. Healthy relationships help us live well. Unless we live as hermits, we interact with other people. In doing so, we risk experiencing conflict, missed communication, bitterness, misunderstanding, incompatible expectation, and disappointment.

"Without loving oneself, it is not possible to love even one's neighbor. Self-hatred is identical with narrow selfishness and, in the end, produces the same horrible isolation, the same desperation."

—Hermann Hesse

Eight Relationship Mistakes

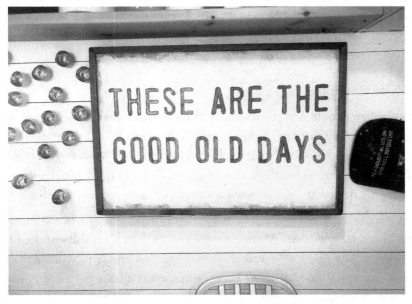

These are the good old days, this sign reminded me of that, Fire Island, 2018

Remember, when you commit you will be challenged. Friendships and relationships require growth and mistakes happen. It's not possible to avoid these mistakes all of the time but knowing about them and being mindful of your responsibility in creating problems is helpful. The three most powerful words to correct any of them is, "I'M SORRY." Remember these words because they will guide you toward creating healthy boundaries.

1. Making offensive comments

When men or women say things to each other that lack tact or sensitivity, just because they feel what they said or did was plain funny, they risk hurting others. It happens to me all the time, as I can lack tact or have a strange sense of humor that doesn't match the situation. For example, I may express judgment after someone tells me something and say something like, "That was stupid!" or "Please, don't be an idiot." While I don't intend it to sound that bad, it is pretty bad, and the other person can take serious offense.

I often think I am being sincere or honest with the other person or trying to help somehow, but they feel that I am being verbally abusive or judging them harshly. Thus, misunderstanding begins.

You can't always predict what another person will or won't feel in a particular situation. So, it is advisable to put yourself in their shoes. Ask yourself if you would like to hear the words you might say before you say them. If you don't like them, why should someone else?

2. Giving solutions

Often, when people want someone to listen to them talk through their problems, we have solutions to the issues bubbling up inside of us. However, when people speak to us about their problems, they mainly look for someone to share their frustrations with, to commiserate. Perhaps, they've had a long and challenging day or are going through a demanding period in their life.

Men and women have different brains. The right and left hemispheres of their brains are different. Women are more verbal on both sides of the brain, whereas men tend to have verbal centers only on the left. Women show a higher emotional literacy, using more words when discussing people, places, or things. Men use fewer words and have less connectivity between their word centers and their memories or feelings. So, it's essential to make space for emotions, sharing, and caring without offering solutions. Sometimes people just need to talk it out.

3. Being judgmental

No one likes to be judged or labeled with, "That's wrong" or "That's low" or "That's ugly" or "This is what I recommend" or "That's just nonsense," etc. The saying that "The head serves to divide the ears" is very appropriate.

If you realize you are constantly judging others for what they do or say, it could help you if you take a break and start looking inside yourself. Recognize that you can be right and alone, or wrong and in a relationship. Relationships are 50/50. Often what you say about others says more about you than them. When you diminish others, you don't make them or yourself any better. You only make yourself look more insecure about your ability to be noncontrolling and nonjudgmental.

It's better to be humble and focus on other people. It's more beneficial to ask questions that help you understand why others do what they do, even if it's not how you do it. Where does judgment impede your relationships? Ask how and where you were judged and if you are doing the same thing to others.

4. Being defensive

No one likes criticism. But if you are always on the defensive, raising walls and barriers to intimacy, using defense mechanisms with others, you cannot have intimate relationships. Look at the word *criticism*. It signifies the hope of making a person better by identifying a better way of being, looking at, or talking about a situation. If you are always on the defensive, you can't allow the wisdom of others to penetrate. As my father would always say, "Only a friend would tell you to comb your hair to look better."

Relationships need to learn how to work with criticism, to move, grow, and evolve. Even a garden of fertile flowers and plants needs a bit of criticism—critiquing—to help it grow. Knowing how to handle criticism could be the most critical skill you can ever acquire. If you spot it, you've probably got it. What is it that you are pushing away because it's not "good enough?" Don't let good be the enemy of perfection.

5. Directing others

When people direct us, it's as if they are in charge of who we are. Does anyone like to be controlled? Certainly not. Yet, a "do this" or "do that" attitude is a part of some people's dialogue. You don't gain friends or influence people if you tell them what to do most of the time. Who made you the boss? Where in your life have you been bossed around? It is more important to learn to collaborate, involve people, ask them questions, listen, and inspire them toward a common purpose. Remember, everyone wants to feel involved somehow, not just as performers but as collaborators.

6. Being a know-it-all

The more we learn, the more we realize we know little. The world contains an enormous wealth of knowledge, ready to be discovered. Life is an infinite learning process. Thinking that you know everything, well, that is a considerable limitation. There is so much of the world to discover beyond books and meeting others. There are over seven billion realities globally, and each person offers something that you can learn from and discover.

When you refuse to consider alternative methods and vehemently defend your way of doing things, it prevents you from connecting with others. An attitude of curiosity helps you be open to different ways of doing things and experimenting with new things in your life. So, breathe in the new and let go of the old.

7. Always complaining

It's okay to complain a little from time to time, but doing it too often pushes people away from you. Whining and complaining too much and too often creates a vortex of negativity that sucks up the energy and focus of positive people around you. You don't want to be an energy vampire.

If you find you are an energy vampire, regularly complaining about someone, something, change your routine. Start by focusing on the positive things. Before you voice a complaint, ask yourself how important it is.

8. Not listening

When someone talks to you, are you present in the conversation? Or do your thoughts and mind go elsewhere?

Mindful listening helps you hear what is being said at the moment and what needs to be heard. It is often the hidden message, the heart's longing just beneath the words. Listen carefully, actively seek to capture the emotions. Hear the message behind their words, in their tone or inflection as it is being said. You can see their eyes water, or a smile come to their face and be surprised to find out how deep the conversation can go.

Toxic People

Sometimes, we can find ourselves in boiling water, especially when dealing with toxic people. The way intelligent people handle toxic people says a lot about their emotional and psychological abilities. They don't let themselves be overcome by the tone or temper that toxic people try to dictate. They know how to define their boundaries and see the impact that others can have on their health.

One of the best things you can do is cultivate your ability to neutralize toxic people, manage your boundaries with them and others they may pollute. Don't get too hot. Allow them to simmer by taking a breath and waiting five to ten seconds before you speak. People treat you how you allow them.

Some sociologists and social psychology experts say that we live in an age charged with toxicity. We are all traumatized implicitly throughout the day as we interact with the world. It's in the news, on television, and in the movies. We get to see violence and toxicity played out in so many ways. We are used to listening and seeing disrespect, anger, and violence, and it is often difficult to know the boundary between what is toxic and what is not.

We live in an era marked by instability and uncertainty, which is reflected in our everyday lives. Tribalism and divisiveness are all around us, and we need to find a quiet place to care for and nourish ourselves with vigilant compassion. It's paradoxical but necessary to identify toxicity and apply a compassionate antidote. Be alert and weed out the issues before they kill what's right.

Hurt people hurt people. They hurt you emotionally, and they also threaten your health. When toxic behavior takes root in a specific context, most people who are part of it end up taking harmful or cynical attitudes.

Many toxic attitudes multiply like a virus in work environments, especially ones where individual productivity is vital. In these dog-eat-dog competitive cultures, distrust, rivalry, envy, and frustration might damage and threaten an organization's systemic well-being.

Toxic people are everywhere. They come in all shapes and sizes—from friends to families or loved ones. People may unwillingly choose to act out thoughts or words that are harmful to their children or their partner. The impact and the damage can be corrosive and scar individuals because of the emotional component or blood bond. Toxic primary relationships can undermine us to the core.

How to manage toxic relationships

The way you mindfully manage toxic relationships depends on several factors. The first simple and obvious consideration is that all unhealthy behavior is illogical. By recognizing that, you won't give so much importance, time, and energy to a series of meaningless actions and words that may erupt from time to time. It's a kind of "I don't mind, and it doesn't matter" attitude. That way, you do not project your discomfort, frustration, and negative emotions onto the other and inflame the situation further. Sounds easy, but it's not. It takes a mindful attitude of conscious compassion. But you don't have to suffer if you don't take it on and are compassionate.

There is a second aspect you cannot underestimate. According to a study by the Department of Clinical Psychology and Biology from Germany's Friedrich Schiller University, prolonged exposure to toxic people or situations can damage brain health.[21] Conscious, compassionate practice is one way to approach these disturbances of the mind.

Being continually subjected to toxicity makes us feel more stressed, anxious, tired, and we cannot concentrate or think clearly. It has a multiplier effect on our bodies by producing more cortisol, fight-or-flight behavior, and less rational thought. Establishing clear boundaries is an essential step toward

---

21 https://pubmed.ncbi.nlm.nih.gov/19846255/

wholeness. Remember, you can wish others well far away from you and give yourself compassionate distancing.

Focus on solutions, not problems

Toxic people in our environment beget a state of constant alertness. It is like seeing a shark or a predator in our midst every day; we live under threat. Remember that intelligent people are more likely to seek solutions to the problem than to focus on toxic behavior. So, step away from the situation and move into rational thought. Focusing on the solution, not the problem, is the answer.

Define boundary lines as soon as possible

We naturally respond in kind to people. Kindness begets kindness. However, when someone is toxic, how should we act to curb their harmful behavior? It's wise to keep in mind that running away is not always worthwhile or that it might be impossible to place a specified distance between the toxic person and yourself.

It's proper to outline boundaries to protect yourself and others. To succeed, you must clarify to the person that their attitudes have consequences, that not everything is allowed, and that some behaviors are destructive and create tension. You must explain from the beginning your limits and boundary lines. You need to be precise. Setting boundaries might sound like, "Please don't yell or talk so loudly if you want me to listen to you."

Proper management of emotions

You need to be fully aware of your emotions. If you feel exhausted or psychologically tired, you must handle that situation. The first thing is to understand that no one has the right to take away your smile or inner calm. The second thing is not to give a vital role to those who do nothing to earn a place in your life. Considering that it might be impossible to distance yourself from toxic people physically, it is best to move away from them emotionally and open your invisible shield to protect yourself. You might use a deflective technique, such as "I really can't hear you right now. Let's talk about this later when you and I are ready to talk."

Cognitive empathy in front of a toxic person

What is cognitive empathy? It is the ability to understand the mechanisms that might work in a toxic person's mind. Maybe their face and stressful dynamics conceal a person whose profile is undiagnosed depression, trauma, or emotional abuse. This person might look at life through a "rearview mirror" and deal with unresolved issues and replay events that happened a long time ago.

Cognitive empathy allows you to understand another's unknown realities without being controlled by emotions that they project on you, based on their own experiences.

This strategy helps us to work out an intelligent way to manage toxic people.

Five Keys to Connecting Mindfully

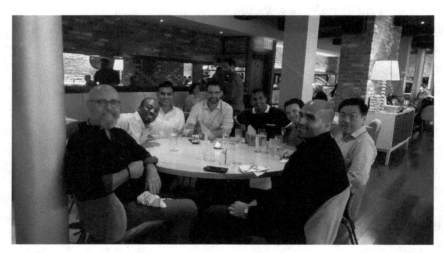

Roundtable of Entrepreneurs, New York, 2018

Communication is the basis of every relationship. Effective communication is a straightforward way to convey information about thought, emotion, and story. It is a specific skill that can be mastered and applied to relationships to create transparency, so there are fewer distortions and more understandings. Fundamental strategies improve relationships and lift effective communication.

1) Listen to what is being said

Focus on the words and what they mean. Avoid not listening and changing the subject to yourself or another topic. When talking with someone about an important issue, refrain from playing with your nails, looking around the room (or worse, the TV), or daydreaming. In conversations, lean toward the other person, make eye contact, and hear what they say before opening your mouth.

2) Avoid blaming

Often, you should just keep your mouth shut when you are caught up in a rage. Whatever you say may sound accusatory when you begin with "You always have…" or "You do not…" Try to use "feel" statements instead, like "I feel it's important that…" Using the word "feel" is always better than "I think." Because no one can argue with how you feel, but they can with how you think. Be mindful, though, feelings and thoughts can change as conditions change.

3) It is essential to calm down (sometimes in solitude) before talking about problems

Some people like to nip things in the bud—and inadvertently do more harm if anger takes over in a discussion. If a situation is heated, calm down. It's helpful to tell your partner that you want a little alone time and discuss the issue later. The longest journey we make in life is between the head and the heart. If it's an important matter, you can rationalize it later with love and compassion.

4) Choose the time and place

Choose a neutral time and a suitable place to discuss your concerns. For example, don't try to discuss a problem before a family trip. It will ruin your mood, and you won't enjoy the journey! Setting an appropriate time and place to discuss issues is vitally important for avoiding negative fallout. I like to use the five-minute share technique, previously mentioned, which sets up the time and place, encourages you to go deep, listen mindfully, and discuss from a "me place."

5) Ask questions and be careful

A reliable rule of thumb is to ask questions like, "How can I help?" or "I'm not sure I understand. What do you mean by that?" or "Where do you want to take that?" Your partner will then feel that you are trying to find a solution to a problem and are sincerely interested in what they think and say.

Mindful Tips

You can have several toxic people around you, and you may even have learned to manage them effectively. And yet, there is something you must not lose sight of even for a moment: your health. That's why you have to give importance to what you eat, how long you rest, and how much time you spend relaxing.

Learning to switch off and not think about those toxic psychological profiles will grant you the quality of life you desire. With a mindful approach, you can develop the tools you need to manage relationships the right way, live a better life, and have a more peaceful, stress-free environment at home and work.

Apply the five tips to improve communication in all your relationships. Remember to focus on solutions and not problems. Give yourself a break if it gets overwhelming, and then return to the relationship. Keep your mindfulness practice going. You will be happier in relationships with yourself and others when you practice love and compassion for your life and the lives of others.

How do you rate yourself?

Relationship: Love, Friends, and Marriage

How would you rate yourself? Do you feel listened to and connected to people you love and care about? What is the quality of your communication with family, friends, and people you work with?

How do you rate yourself on a scale of 1 (low) to 5 (high)?

Where are you?

1	2	3	4	5

Where do you want to be?

1	2	3	4	5

Why did you choose this number?

_____

_____

_____

What changes could you make to help you get there?

_____

_____

_____

Source: Personal Health Inventory –

Veterans Affairs. https://www.va.gov/WHOLEHEALTH/docs/10-773_PHI_May2020.pdf

ASPIRATION

Chapter 8

ASPIRATION

Learning and Growing

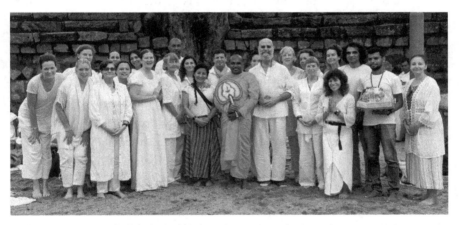

*On Pilgrimage, with Dr. Miles Neale and other pilgrims, Sri
Lanka 2019, courtesy of Jordan Harvey, Photographer*

THIS LAST STRATEGY is perhaps the most important. Aspiration involves the integration and growth of all of the other approaches outlined so far. Aspiration gets set into motion when we improve and raise ourselves, our consciousness, above our current condition or circumstance. What happens when we want to achieve something more—have peace of mind, a better body, a connection with our spirits, better sleep? We get inspired and ready to work, do the work, perspire, manifest, and realize our inner and outward manifestations.

❧

People who aspire to be better, to improve themselves, are focused on self-improvement. "To aspirate" also means "to breathe," mainly "to breathe in or inhale." How did *aspiration* come to mean "ambition or the will to succeed, improve, and do better?" It was once believed that our breath was our soul or spirit. The Latin root word *spīritus* means (breath) and the word *spīrāre* means (breathe). It is no coincidence that the words conspire, expire, inspire, perspire, respiration, respire, spirit, and transpire all involve the rising, falling, or exchange or giving of breath to something or taking it away.[22] That might explain why we talk about *breathing life into something* or *rising with energy and ideas to invigorate the spirit for something.*

Our breath fills us with an inner urge to create something for ourselves. We are inspired, creators. If we nurture ourselves and are kind to ourselves in mind, speech, and body, we apply ourselves and look to the outer world for aspiration to move forward and upward. If we are not nurturing and kind internally, we can perspire and sweat the small stuff; and as a result, we don't rise to find our inspiration or the aspiration to move into the world.

When we "sweat the small stuff" with worry and upset, our energy drains into a downward spiral. There is no wind in our sails, the meaning in our lives may be gone, and we may no longer find purpose. This is depression, which, when long-lasting, can become a severe health condition. It can cause a person to suffer enormously and function poorly at work, school, and in the family.

Depression can even lead to suicide. Close to 800,000 people die from suicide every year. It is the second leading cause of death of those in the age range fifteen to twenty-nine. A study from the Perelman School of Medicine at the University of Pennsylvania found that a breathing-based meditation can help ease severe depression in people who did not fully respond to antidepressant treatments.[23]

Many believe that our breath expresses the most profound longing of our spirits and souls. The breath's energy inspires us to balance our inner world, and we aspire to be the change we wish to see in the world. This is what is meant by breathing life into something. In our search for balance, to integrate mind, body, and spirit, the breath calls us to move, change, and let go of old worn-out ideas and adopt a fresh way of being.

---

22 https://www.dailywritingtips.com/the-latin-word-for-breathe-inspired-many-english-terms/

23 https://www.sciencedaily.com/releases/2016/11/161122182357.htm

This chapter looks at self-improvement and how mindfulness and integration of body, mind, and spirit inspire us to show up for our hopes, dreams, and ambitions. To achieve something—to aspire for a life beyond the day-to-day normality—we need to be the heroes of our own stories. However, the adventure of a lifetime finds many of us caught between the proverbial rock and a hard place. We sweat and perspire at the prospect of change and upheaval, so we do nothing to change our old stories. Our dreams die inside, and so do we. We may start with the best of intentions, but then we get caught between the shadows of comparison and despair. *Who am I to want to be better? Why don't I just settle for less?* We numb ourselves and instead live lives of quiet desperation.

So, what do we do, and how do we break out of the restrictions, resistance, fears, and uncertainties that hold us back?

We fill life with opportunities to grow, improve, accentuate what is positive, and reduce the negative things in our lives. Yet, the path is not always clear. Some people think it's impossible to rise above negativity and break free; they feel helpless and defeated and don't heed the call to change.

Change is challenging. If we want to change, we must be prepared to meet the challenge of leaving our comfort zones and be ready to risk it all. The path of the hero is fraught with challenges and disappointment. There are many enemies, ghosts, and demons to fight along the way to transformation.

Science shows us we can build a new neural network that will be our new cognitive pathway. We can visualize and develop new relationships with people, places, and things. By being in contact with our spirits, our souls, and our psyches' most intimate longings, we can materialize a new reality for ourselves. Mindfully getting up close, face-to-face, with our self-limiting belief systems, we can change our stories.

Stepping up to the challenge, confronting our belief systems, may be painful, though, as change often requires us to look at and deal with traumas. But, by consistently cleaning, clearing, and challenging our narratives and self-limiting beliefs, we can weed them out and seed, feed, and grow new self-affirming, virtuous deeds. And then, we can act to materialize the new reality. We seed new beliefs when we work differently and encourage ourselves to break away from the old self-limiting belief systems. We repattern ourselves to form new realities, behaviors, and ways of being different on emotional and material levels.

Self-improvement asks us to consistently clean the windshields of the mind's eye to see the world differently. And self-improvement requires us to wipe clean our perceptions and self-limiting chatter in order to recognize and choose a different way of being and becoming. With focus, concentration, and effort, we can choose to respond rather than merely react to thoughts, perceptions, emotions, or meanderings that change moment by moment.

I recommend starting by having a dialogue with yourself. Ask yourself every type of open question you can think of to understand your inner working dialogue better, questions like these.

Why do I do what I do? Who gave me my beliefs? What is it about the situation that triggers me emotionally and elicits automatic routine behaviors and responses? What do I do because of those triggers? Can I recognize and adjust my actions?

Take a Mindful Pause to bring awareness to your thoughts, emotions, and sensations, to acknowledge and choose new behaviors.

Skillful Means

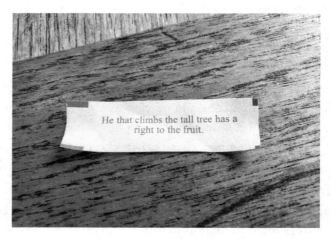

He that climbs the tall tree has a right to the fruit.

Sometimes it's right in front of us,
fortune cookie wisdom, 2016

Mindfulness can offer us skills to manage our emotions, resilience, empathy, adaptability, and creativity. Transversal skills, or soft skills, are helpful in our private lives and our professions.

Research has shown that technical knowledge and emotional intelligence help establish us in life and profession. But managing emotions is an essential everyday requirement to live life fully. Managing your feelings means recognizing the good, bad, and indifferent feelings that arise and giving them a name. Naming emotions is called emotional literacy. When you can tag and bag them, you can understand the information they contain and link them to the causes, conditions, and messages or triggers that started them. You can use emotions to better understand the world around you, learn about the causes and conditions for your feelings, traumas, and patterns, and excavate and rebuild your life. With a compassionate intention, you can change your story and change your life.

Being able to sense unpleasant emotions emerging helps you calm the tsunamis that trigger you. With emotional literacy, you understand your stories, triggers, ups, downs, and how you look at the world and relate to others. Mindfulness allows you to have a more full-hearted life, to realize that it is not about how good or bad life is; it's about your ability to accept, integrate, and open to a bigger, broader life based on inspiration and aspiration.

With a mindful approach, you can wake up every day as if it's a new day, breathe the air, recognize, and choose your waking moments with acceptance. With an inhalation, you remember to be the person you want to be and let go of any negativity with an exhalation. You rejoin those pieces of your life that fragmented overnight. You become present to your potential in the early daylight hours, using a calm, clear concentration that connects intention with what is essential. *What is vital to living life with a positive forward momentum? How can I be present to my aspirational possibilities in the present?*

Letting go of the past and acting in a way that looks to understand, be understood, and understand each moment is an essential requirement of having a presence. When we stop looking outside for affirmation and look inside for guidance, we find our inner voice, like a GPS guide, for a direction free of society's distractions.

Throughout the COVID pandemic, so many of us have learned that we can find ourselves at a crossroads needing to choose between what we have and what we need. Yet, regardless of what we have or the situation we find ourselves in, we can be challenged by other voices from our jobs, families, relationships, or inner critic and judge.

Use mindfulness to get in touch with the inner guide to get on the right path. These three tools have helped me to power up in my life.

Three fundamental tools for listening to your voice:

1. Self-compassion

To understand self-compassion, think about compassion. To be compassionate to others means listening to them by putting yourself in their shoes, so you can understand what is bothering them and help. When you see yourself in others, you find compassion for yourself. You back away from the vehicle of your own life and start to see how you are not alone. With that perspective, you can offer wishes to yourself and others for wellness, peace, happiness, and freedom from suffering.

You need to know what triggers you, what narratives you create, how you respond to those old stories, and then change those stories and your life. By adopting an attitude of gratitude and nonattachment, you can find and create novel ways of being in situations and thus recognize and choose different outcomes.

2. Gratitude

The greatest gift you can give to life is a sense of gratitude. I like to say that what we appreciate, appreciates in value. There are different ways to learn how to generate appreciation. I keep a gratitude diary, which helps me to recognize what I have that I can be thankful for at every moment of every day.

Much of the happiness you can enjoy lies within you, but it is not free. You need to activate happiness, just as you start electricity with a switch. There's a choice, and gratitude switches it on; ingratitude switches it off. In between satisfaction and dissatisfaction is a space, which is open to human potential. You get to choose how you light up your life or darken it, whether your path goes forward, grows, stands still, or withers.

3. Meditation

Self-compassion, gratitude, and meditation are three tools that have helped me dive into questions of needs, wants, and desires for living the kind of life I want. Meditation is the primary tool I use for living my life, my secret weapon. Every morning it helps me introduce space into my life—into what some call the *gap* or the *margins* in life—to make room for "*the me I want to be.*" Meditation stretches my reaction time to stimulus. So, I can measure my response, check in with my best intentions and respond appropriately. I can align my actions with my aspirational values for love and compassion.

Self-improvement develops when you develop your insights into what is missing in your life. Introspection creates conscious awareness of who you are and what you wish to be in the world based on what you value. With this awareness, you find inspiration to move beyond your current conditions, to lift your circumstances to another level.

Being aware of your thinking, seeing how you are with or without judgment offers you the ability to be an active participant in your development—you can know and see yourself through the awareness of your becoming. You come face-to-face with your critics, external and internal. With effort, concentration, and devotion to being present, you repeatedly return to the questions that help you benefit others and yourself without running, hiding, or going numb. *Why am I here? What is my passion? What can I do to be of benefit?*

Self-improvement is a journey. It's also a metaphor for seeing and being present again and again, as if for the first time, day after day, week after week, month after month. Each time, your journey has a departure, an arrival, and adventures and nuances in the middle. It is a continual cycle you go through every day as you wake up and later sleep. Every day you experience new encounters, unknown places, new people, fresh smells, and unique flavors during this journey and alternative ways (perceptions) for looking at yourself and others.

Whether you are out and about in the world or at home, this journey is sometimes long, sometimes tortuous, sometimes tiring, sometimes beautiful, sometimes ugly, and often unknown. You can live it with awareness, awe, and a determination to discover new parts of yourself, new opportunities, and new resources—or you can refuse the journey and sit still, numb, ignorant of the options to experience everything that life has to offer.

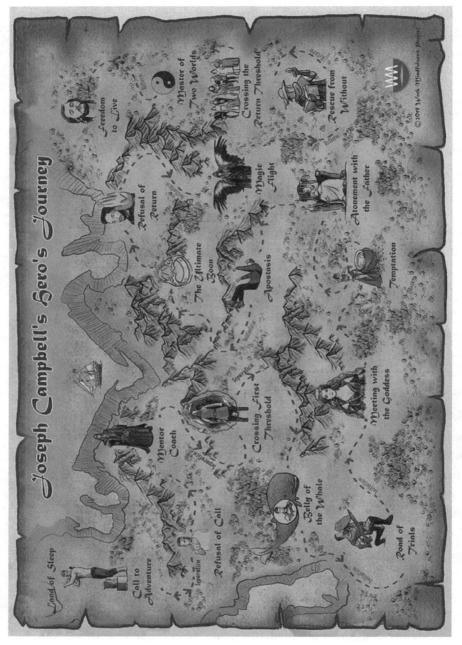

The Hero's Journey Map, designed by Workmindfulness.com

The Hero's Journey

The illustrated graphic on the previous page is based on Joseph Campbell's work on The Hero's Journey. The graphic depicts an aspirational journey, what is called a monomyth. The hero of the story (which is you, me, every man, woman and child) decides wake-up to life. Previously, life had no energy it was like being in the land of sleep. The hero decides to live a life that does not stagnate, that has growth, change, and transformation. Joseph Campbell, an American professor of literature at Sarah Lawrence College, who worked in comparative mythology and comparative religion, called it The Hero's Journey. It is the journey that each of us takes to hear the call for our soul's longing, calling for itself to be heard and recognized. We yearn for change and transformation, but many of us don't heed the call. We go back to sleep, dulling our senses because of fear or doubt. [24]

The three Cs

The three Cs for living an aspirational journey are Courage, Connection, and Change.

Courage

Courage is necessary because the journey involves research, discovery, and willingness to rediscover who you are repeatedly. It requires you to wake up from the land of sleep (the need to be numb) and move away from what is easy. You act with courage and presence in what is happening from moment to moment. Listen to your heart's longing and do what is necessary to get unstuck.

Courage requires courageousness because getting unstuck does not feel pleasant. You can feel lost, incomplete, frustrated, anxious, and unhappy because of emotional blocks and habits that lock you into causes and conditions. You may not always be aware of these inner emotional blocks. A path of personal growth facilitates awareness to understand your personal stories, rights, and wrongs.

---

24   https://en.wikipedia.org/wiki/Hero%27s_journey

Be aware of an issue or emotional upset, decipher your choices, needs, and emotions. Using a process of self-inquiry and self-knowledge, you actively listen to your stories and excuses, with a more detailed awareness of what you wish to change. It's important to always ask yourself, *If nothing changes, if I stay where I am, will I be happier with what I am doing than if I change?*

Connection

Connection is necessary because you must have the inner resolve and strength to carry on, with faith in yourself and

your vision for change. The big wake-up moments occur in life when you recognize something needs to change. What is it that is missing? What will help you to connect more to your life and breath? It may be the death of a loved one, the loss of a job, a wife, a husband, a family member, a health diagnosis, or a job promotion. You wake up one day and say that there must be something more in life! You say *I need to find out what life is all about, beyond the walls of my home, the borders of my town, the land and system I know!* You connect to your inner power and resolve to move forward.

God moves mountains, but we need to bring the shovel. I have started over several times in my life, taken stock of my life, and started adventures in a new life, with a shovel by my side and faith and connection to a higher purpose. What is your quest or purpose? What is driving you to say goodbye to the old and move into the new? A new life requires that you leave behind people, places, and things. You have to be connected to a higher purpose, to find the energy and courage to move forward.

Change

You must be the change you wish to see in the world. You cannot grow old and die without changing, but change requires a commitment to move forward. It requires the capacity to generate opportunities to fill the space, the inherent feeling of emptiness, and discomfort that can feel inexhaustible. The hole in the soul can have you move from being a consumer of material things and leisure to being a consumer of therapies, techniques, or disciplines as you seek to fill the emptiness of your life. You cannot circumvent your soul's longing with some New Age recipe or religious dogma.

You must be your healer and go deep to discover and illuminate your inner challenges on this path of discovery. There are no fast-food personal growth solutions to understand your fears or doubts. Doing your work is essential on the road to self-realization. You must face your nature, what you've created and inherited, and deal with it. You must uproot it, unmask your true identity, and unhook yourself from the traumas that bind you. By doing that, you can open your heart and mind to the possibility of changing your circumstances and relationships to people, places, and things.

Personal growth requires that you undertake a course of awareness about reality. Focus on your core beliefs, relationships with others, and future opportunities, based on the behaviors, thoughts, and feelings that rightly or wrongly form your perceptions of the world. Be centered in your meditation, your intentions, and plant the seeds of compassion and care necessary for growth to change your story. Focus on yourself, those close to you and in need, and those you don't know personally but know are suffering (COVID patients, for example). Plant seeds of compassion and wish for change and well-being.

By practicing mindfulness, you can generate greater awareness for your every breath and every moment that passes. You can be more present to whatever life brings you in the present. You can exercise your conscious awareness of the love and compassion you have for your own life and for the possibility of a future created from the seeds of potential you nourish every waking moment. With effort and concentration, you can develop awareness for the present moment by consistently bringing yourself back to the present.

Benefits of Inspiration/Aspiration and Self-Improvement

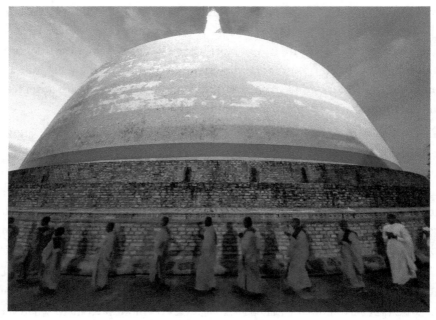

On Pilgrimage, monks, circumambulating at Thuparama Seya-SriLanka, 2019

We move off automatic pilot, that state of boredom when tasks are mindless routines, and generate the following benefits:

- Increased concentration
- A sense of purpose
- Reduced time in reactive mode
- Better control of thoughts, emotions, and behaviors
- More enjoyment of the present moment
- More profound relaxation, improved breathing, regulation of blood pressure, and strengthening of the immune system
- Higher quality relationships with others

Mindfulness can help you find inspiration and aspiration by:

- Opening you to acceptance of any situation and emotion, even though it may be unpleasant. What you resist persists, but with mindfulness, you can step back, recognize the problem, accept it, investigate it, nurture its processing, and cool your overreactions.

- Helping you to release or let go of things. Even knowing how to detach from other people or situations, when necessary, can be tricky. You need to remove your expectations.

- Generating an essential curiosity or a beginner's mind, the same as children spontaneously do. By opening up to your nature, curiosity helps you understand internal and external worlds that move you.

- Encouraging you to experience gratitude, which is the most extraordinary form of worship in my estimation. Having an appreciation for the simple things in life, like the water you drink or bathe in, and feeling grateful for the little things in life, like breathing, eating, and sleeping, are qualities you develop over time. A grateful mind is a soft pillow.

Staying fully attentive involves perceiving your emotions and moods without judging them, noticing what reactions arise, and how feelings, attitudes, and perspectives continually change during the day. By acting consciously, concentrating on each activity, and being present and attentive to your needs and those of the people around you, you can share, care for, and have heightened enjoyment and quality in your day.

Every day try to apply the following techniques:

- **Breathing-based meditation**: work on conscious breathing as a basis for physical and mental relaxation.

- **Walking meditation**: adjust your breathing to the steps you take while walking and focus on the sensations the act of walking produces in you—posture, body weight, the position of your feet, and balance.

- **Body scan**: base this on conscious attention to your body, muscle relaxation, and mental state.

- **Full attention in everyday life**: savor your food, contemplate and observe images, listen to music, laugh, smile, and unlearn automatic-pilot behaviors in your daily tasks.

Five mindfulness exercises to inspire

These exercises will help you create an attitude of gratitude for life. You don't want to memorize activities, but you want to adopt a way of facing the events in your daily life. Think of your body as an outer vehicle that will help you navigate the world. These practices are the engine, fuel, and steering wheel to help you get where you want to go.

1. Mindfulness in a single minute

Start with a minute and then increase your practice time to fifteen or twenty minutes a day. Because it is only a minute, you can practice mindfulness anywhere during the day or even at night before going to bed if you have trouble sleeping.

Practice: Breathe in, breathe out, be aware of your breath, the rise and fall of your chest and stomach, the feeling of the breath at your nose, and the awareness of all your senses (eyes, ears, nose, mouth, air on the skin, the body, and the thoughts). Repeat.

2. Breathing for landing here and now

This exercise is ideal for turning off the autopilot. Focusing your attention on the present moment stops the constant flow of thoughts, memories, images, or ideas. It is ideal for discharging accumulated tension simply. Focus your attention on your breathing.

Practice: Take a soft, deep, and constant inhalation through your nose. Fill your lungs and belly. Immediately release the air through your mouth with intensity but without forcing your throat. When you notice a distraction (which is normal), observe what caught your attention, then return to your breath again.

3. Mindfulness breakfast

We usually get up in the morning on autopilot—wake up, check our phones, get out of bed, shower, dress, have breakfast, brush our teeth, and go off to another day of work.

With this exercise, you break harmful habits by practicing mindfulness in the morning, so you face the day in another way.

Practice: Sit in a quiet place, turn off the TV, and switch your phone to silent mode. It's about having no distractions. When you have your breakfast, focus your attention on the flavors, smells, and taste of the food or drink. In this way, you are paying attention to the present moment.

4. Attending to the sounds of the moment

Consciously observe the sounds that occur in your environment. When listening to sounds, related thoughts and feelings arise. Try to just experience the sound and silence, without thinking, letting the sound waves wash over your body, feeling and experiencing them.

Practice: Listen to the sounds in your environment. Hear them as they happen without identifying them, judging them as pleasant or unpleasant, or thinking about them. With no effort, observe the sounds and external perceptions, then let them go. Watch how the sounds change and notice how your mind moves toward distraction. Observe the gap between the sounds, then return to listening to the sounds, relying only on the breath at that moment.

5. Body scan

With this exercise, you get in touch with your body's experience without judging it, rejecting unpleasant sensations, or holding on to pleasant ones.

Practice: Sit in a comfortable position with a straight back, although it is also possible to adopt a lying position. Close your eyes, pay attention to your breath, and journey through your body.

It's advisable to be guided for this type of meditation. Signing up for the mobile app called "Insight Timer" is a great idea, and look for guided meditations (including mine) that focus on body scanning. See the resources in the Appendix.

Mindful Tips

In this chapter, we've looked at how you can change and grow with inspiration and aspiration. In the past year, because of COVID, you've had to grow and stretch a lot. You've had to find inspiration in the quiet moments of prayer and solitude. You've discovered aspiration in stories of hope and recovery; so many people have been impacted.

Growth requires that you change, on the inside and outside—the people, places, things, conscious attitudes, thoughts, and patterns. You are constantly evolving through small acts of courage and commitment. Whether you are ready for it, change will challenge you and the very things you know and love. But it will also help you to understand yourself better. It will ask you to try alternative ways of being, open your awareness to life, and transform yourself.

Lean into change because it will help you to:

- Improve your relationship with your life and the lives of others
- Give you belief in yourself and your abilities
- Strengthen your self-esteem
- Improve psychological well-being
- Identify and enhance your resources
- Promote your autonomy
- Facilitate your decision-making skills
- Develop more practical and functional strategies
- Be resilient

Psychological distress (existential, emotional, relational, or familial) can negatively affect your daily life by causing psychophysical symptoms of stress, anxiety, depression, phobias, panic attacks, aggression, and sleep disorders. Distress impacts your psychophysical well-being. With mindfulness, it is possible to find inspiration during tough times and analyze the difficulty. You can find inspiration in simple things, set achievable goals, and find your aspiration to work and create in the world.

By incorporating mindfulness into your life, self-esteem becomes an essential self-supporting tool during distress. By providing yourself with a welcoming and nonjudgmental listening space for your inner critic, you allow your psyche to discover, accept, and heal emotions, suffering, and traumas that may have been repressed or buried.

With mindfulness, we facilitate an awareness of the narrative and cognitive processes in our lives that help us pave a path to change. The change we wish to see requires understanding the old story as we take the first step toward a new story. We look at opportunities for personal growth and emotional well-being—a path of personal growth that helps us to love and be here now.

How do you rate yourself?

Aspiration: *Learning and growing.*

Developing abilities and talents. Balancing responsibilities where you live, volunteer, and work.

Rate yourself on a scale of 1 (low) to 5 (high).

Where are you?

1	2	3	4	5

Where do you want to be?

1	2	3	4	5

Why did you choose this number?

_____

_____

_____

What changes could you make to help you get there?

_____

_____

_____

Source: Personal Health Inventory –

Veterans Affairs. https://www.va.gov/WHOLEHEALTH/docs/10-773_PHI_May2020.pdf

Appendix

The appendix contains various sections that you can use in your daily life to put these eight strategies into practice to have a more balanced life. Use it as a resource and access it for practical help.

You'll find an inventory you can use to assess your balance, and there are suggestions on what you can do next. Finally, you'll discover some website links and meditation scripts that you can use for various situations.

Eight Strategies Assessment

In this section, you can assess your life's balance using the same measures that you used at the ends of chapters 1 through 8.

You can take the challenge to grab hold of your life and transform any suffering into joy and happiness. Knowing your health goals may not be a simple task. Yet, it is an essential step toward reaching your full potential. Look over the eight areas that make up this book. See how you are doing in each one of the eight strategic areas.

Please review each of the chapters to help you create your life balance program. Your life is an ongoing activity from dusk to dawn. Each day you need to show up as your best self. Every experience you have can influence your physical and emotional health, your mind, body and spiritual health, and well-being. The human body and mind have tremendous healing abilities that you can strengthen.

Find Balance Inventory

What matters to you in your life? What brings you a sense of joy and happiness? Place a circle on the scales of 1–5 to show where you feel you are.

Physical well-being

1	2	3	4	5

Miserable   Great

Mental/Emotional well-being

1	2	3	4	5

Miserable   Great

Life: How is your day-to-day life?

1	2	3	4	5

Miserable   Great

For each area below, consider where you are now and where you would like to be. All of the measurements are essential. In the "Where are you?" box, briefly write the reasons you chose your number. In the "Where do you want to be?" box, note some changes that might make this area better for you. Some areas are strongly interconnected, so you may notice some of your answers are the same. You do not have to write in every area or do it all at one time. You might start with the easier ones and return to the harder ones later. It is okay just to circle the numbers.

Mind: *Strengthen and Focus.*

Tapping into the power of your mind can help you to heal and manage discomfort. By using the breath and body scanning techniques, you can recognize, accept, investigate, and accept your situation or change the outcome.

Rate yourself on a scale of 1 (low) to 5 (high).

Where are you?

1	2	3	4	5

Where do you want to be?

1	2	3	4	5

Why did you choose this number?

_____

_____

_____

What changes could you make to help you get there?

_____

_____

_____

Source: Personal Health Inventory –

Veterans Affairs. https://www.va.gov/WHOLEHEALTH/docs/10-773_PHI_May2020.pdf

Body: *Energy and Flexibility.*

Are you active? Do you move your muscles and include movement and physical activities, like walking, dancing, gardening, sports, lifting weights, yoga, cycling, swimming, and working out in a gym, into your daily, weekly routines?

Rate yourself on a scale of 1 (low) to 5 (high).

Where are you?

1	2	3	4	5

Where do you want to be?

1	2	3	4	5

Why did you choose this number?

_____

_____

_____

What changes could you make to help you get there?

_____

_____

_____

Source: Personal Health Inventory –

Veterans Affairs. https://www.va.gov/WHOLEHEALTH/docs/10-773_PHI_May2020.pdf

Spirit: *Growing and Connecting.*

Having a sense of purpose and meaning in your life, feeling connected to something larger than yourself, and finding strength in difficult times.

Rate yourself on a scale of 1 (low) to 5 (high).

Where are you?

| 1 | 2 | 3 | 4 | 5 |

Where do you want to be?

| 1 | 2 | 3 | 4 | 5 |

Why did you choose this number?

_____

_____

_____

What changes could you make to help you get there?

_____

_____

_____

Source: Personal Health Inventory –

Veterans Affairs. https://www.va.gov/WHOLEHEALTH/docs/10-773_PHI_May2020.pdf

Fuel: *Eat and Nourish.*

I am eating healthy, balanced meals with plenty of fruits and vegetables each day, drinking enough water, and limiting sodas, sweetened drinks, and alcohol.

Rate yourself on a scale of 1 (low) to 5 (high).

Where are you?

1	2	3	4	5

Where do you want to be?

1	2	3	4	5

Why did you choose this number?

_____

_____

_____

What changes could you make to help you get there?

_____

_____

_____

Source: Personal Health Inventory –

Veterans Affairs. https://www.va.gov/WHOLEHEALTH/docs/10-773_PHI_May2020.pdf

Recharge: *Sleep and Refresh.*

Getting enough rest, relaxation, and sleep to feel energized during the day.

Rate yourself on a scale of 1 (low) to 5 (high).

Where are you?

1	2	3	4	5

Where do you want to be?

1	2	3	4	5

Why did you choose this number?

_____

_____

_____

What changes could you make to help you get there?

_____

_____

_____

Source: Personal Health Inventory –

Veterans Affairs. https://www.va.gov/WHOLEHEALTH/docs/10-773_PHI_May2020.pdf

Environment: *Physical and Emotional* .

Having comfortable, healthy spaces where you work and live—the quality of the lighting, color, air, and water: decreasing unpleasant clutter, noises, and smells.

Rate yourself on a scale of 1 (low) to 5 (high).

Where are you?

| 1 | 2 | 3 | 4 | 5 |

Where do you want to be?

| 1 | 2 | 3 | 4 | 5 |

Why did you choose this number?

_____

_____

_____

What changes could you make to help you get there?

_____

_____

_____

Source: Personal Health Inventory –

Veterans Affairs. https://www.va.gov/WHOLEHEALTH/docs/10-773_PHI_May2020.pdf

Relationships: *Love, Friends, and Marriage.*

Do you feel listened to and connected to people you love and care about? What is the quality of your communication with family, friends, and people you work with?

Rate yourself on a scale of 1 (low) to 5 (high).

Where are you?

1	2	3	4	5

Where do you want to be?

1	2	3	4	5

Why did you choose this number?

_____

_____

_____

What changes could you make to help you get there?

_____

_____

_____

Source: Personal Health Inventory –

Veterans Affairs. https://www.va.gov/WHOLEHEALTH/docs/10-773_PHI_May2020.pdf

Aspiration: *Learning and Growing.*

Developing abilities and talents. Balancing responsibilities where you live, volunteer, and work.

Rate yourself on a scale of 1 (low) to 5 (high).

Where are you?

1	2	3	4	5

Where do you want to be?

1	2	3	4	5

Why did you choose this number?

_____

_____

_____

What changes could you make to help you get there?

_____

_____

_____

Source: Personal Health Inventory –

Veterans Affairs. https://www.va.gov/WHOLEHEALTH/docs/10-773_PHI_May2020.pdf

Reflections

Which areas of the inventory had a low score? If you have a specific area that presents resistance to you, go back and reread the chapter.

Each area of resistance represents an opportunity for you to grow. So, meet the challenge with commitment. Start slowly and work on the area that will offer you the most balance.

I invite you now to reflect on the following questions, given your answers to the previous assessment. What are you willing to commit to? Remember, the nature of commitment is a challenge.

What is your vision of your best possible health?

_____

_____

_____

_____

_____

What kinds of changes can you make?

_____

_____

_____

_____

_____

_____

What would your life look like then?

_____

_____

_____

_____

_____

_____

What kinds of activities would you be doing?

_____

_____

_____

_____

_____

Are there any areas you would like to work on? Where might you start?

_____

_____

_____

_____

_____

Where To from Here?

The journey we have taken together throughout this book has, I hope, generated some momentum, so you feel supported to do your very best to find balance in an unbalanced world.

At this stage, you probably still feel as if you are pretty new at practicing some of the habits outlined in each of the eight areas. You may not feel confident or ready to go it alone. That is entirely normal and understandable! But it is also an opportunity to make these practices your truth and integrate them more fully into your life.

If you keep in mind your commitment and why you have been cultivating this mindfulness habit, it will balance your life. Hopefully, you have caught some rich glimpses during your practice over these weeks and have seen why this is worthwhile, and why it is essential for you to live your life mindfully. It is like planting a seed of intention to live your life in a more meaningful way. It is never easy to know how this seed will germinate, and when, and how the plant will be nourished and grow. It may feel that the seed is lying dormant. It is only waiting for the right time to be reawakened.

We continue to be beginners and to learn something new about our lives. With each difficulty, we can learn to become less reactive and kinder to ourselves. If we can keep the practices going, focused on the mind, body, spirit, fuel, and recharging, we will find the reward. We will deepen our experiences, which will truly enrich our lives. We will connect with others in relationships, our environment, and inspiration, and we will rise with aspiration.

Most of all, I recommend you continue the formal practice of mindfulness, in whatever form suits you the best, alongside informal practices integrated into your everyday life. These are like the two wings of a bird: they support and strengthen one another.

It may help you see if there is a local practice group, meditation class, or teacher who can support you with your practice, sustain inspiration, and help you overcome difficulties if they arise. If there is nothing available locally, perhaps you have a few friends or colleagues who would like to meet and practice together, using one of the popular apps over Zoom?

Thirty-five mindfulness tips

1. Bring awareness to your breath and body when you wake up in the morning, take a few conscious breaths, and practice half-smiling before getting out of bed.

2. From time to time during the day, bring awareness to your posture and how you transition between body movements, especially when you sit down to eat.

3. Bring awareness to your breathing at various times of the day. Choose to take a few conscious breaths, following the breath in and out. Count ten full breaths and then start again.

4. Use natural mindfulness triggers during the day to return your attention to the present moment: when the phone rings, pass through doorways, stop at traffic lights, when a sound comes into your awareness. Use these moments to breathe, experience your bodily sensations, and feel your feet on the ground.

5. When you eat or drink, bring awareness to the process of stopping, tasting, sensing, and nourishing yourself. Count to ten for each chew before you swallow.

6. Bring awareness to your body sensations as you go about your day, feeling the touch of air on your skin, the parts of the body in contact with the ground, the movement of your limbs as you walk, garden, run, stretch, or lift weights.

7. Notice when you are rushing or hurrying. Bring awareness to your state of mind, emotions, and body sensations in these moments. Notice if tension is arising. See if there is a possibility of choosing a different stance. Whenever possible, do just one thing at a time. Enjoy the present moment!

8. When you find yourself waiting or queuing for something, use those moments as valuable opportunities to stop and tune into your feelings. If you are feeling impatient, bring awareness to that. Don't turn away from your feelings but look at them with curiosity.

9. Bring awareness to rising tensions in your body during the day or check periodically for pressure in your most vulnerable spots. Use this uneasiness as a barometer for your stress level. When possible, breathe into the uneasiness, and let go.

10. Continue to choose daily activities that you can conduct consciously with mindful attention: brushing your teeth, showering, washing, getting dressed. Pay full attention to what you are doing, and when your mind wanders, bring it back. Stay present with your presence of mind.

11. Bring awareness to your communication patterns: talking, listening, and periods of silence; notice your states of mind during these activities. Especially, notice the silence and the sounds in between the silence.

12. Try to be more present during the moments of your life: feeling the breeze on your skin as your walk, noticing the small flower that is growing out of the crack in the wall, the call of the wild geese flying overhead as they start their long journey homeward.

13. Practice turning your mind toward a more positive frame: reflect on everything you feel grateful for today, reflect on the positive moments and what has gone well.

14. Before falling asleep at night, bring awareness to your breathing and your body sensations for at least five full breaths, all the way in and out. These deep breaths will activate the parasympathetic nervous system and help you to rest.

15. Take five to thirty minutes in the morning to be quiet and meditate: sit or lie down and be with yourself, gaze out of the window, listen to the sounds of nature, or take a slow, quiet walk. Be with yourself and remember what is important to you.

16. While your car is warming up, take a quiet minute to pay attention to your breathing. Before you put your foot on the gas, remember the brake; you don't always have to go forward. You can stop, pause, check for traffic, and then proceed.

17. When you drive, be aware of any body tension, your hands on the steering wheel, shoulders, stomach, etc. Consciously work at releasing and dissolving any tensions. Feel what it is like to be relaxed.

18. Decide not to play the radio and be with yourself. Be aware of where you are in the car and how the world is moving around you. Be present where you are now, and let that be enough for the moment. Your GPS is in control.

19. Experiment with driving a little slower than you might usually. Take your foot off of the gas and go in the slower lane.

20. Pay attention to your breathing, the sky, and the trees, or the quality of your mind when you stop at the traffic lights. What does the environment outside look like? What can you appreciate?

21. Take a moment to orient yourself to your workday. If you are driving to work, once you park your car, walk across the car park to step into your life: know where you are and where you are going.

22. While sitting at your desk, computer, etc., pay attention to your bodily sensations and consciously attempt to relax and rid yourself of excess tension. Remember to be present to whatever you are working on and focus your attention on your breath.

23. Use your breaks to relax rather than simply pausing from your work. For instance, instead of having coffee, a cigarette, or reading, take a short walk outside. Go around the block, look at the sky and the trees, and be aware of your feet as you walk.

24. At lunch, changing your environment can be helpful. If you take your lunch, or work at home, go to another room. Try eating at different times and being aware of the sensations of hunger or satiation.

25. Close your door (if you have one) and take some time to relax consciously. Close your eyes and breathe, counting your breaths and letting go of the day behind you and ahead.

26. Decide to STOP for one to three minutes every hour during the workday. Become aware of your breathing and bodily sensations, allowing your mind to settle. You are not a human doing; you are a human being.

27. Use simple cues in your environment as reminders to center yourself—the telephone ringing, sitting at the computer, bathroom breaks, walks, etc.

28. Take some time at lunchtime or other moments in the day to speak with close friends or associates. Choose topics that are not necessarily work-related and be aware of when it's just surface talk (weather, sports, news), which is okay.

29. Choose to eat one or two lunches per week in silence. Use this time

to eat slowly and be with yourself. Focus your attention on chewing your food, slowly tasting each bite before you swallow.

30. At the end of the workday, try retracing the day's activities. Acknowledge and congratulate yourself for what you've accomplished, and then make a list for tomorrow. You've done enough for today!

31. As you walk to the car, pay attention. Breathe in the air, feel the cold or warmth of your body. Can you be open to and accept these environmental conditions and body sensations rather than resisting them? Listen to the sounds. Can you walk without feeling rushed? What happens when you slow down?

32. While your car is warming up, sit quietly and consciously transition from work to home, from the store to home, from one place to another. Just take a moment to be and enjoy it for a moment.

33. While driving, notice if you are rushing. What does it feel like? What could you do about this or that? Remember, you've got more control than you might imagine.

34. When you pull into the driveway at home, take a minute to orient yourself to being with your family and entering your home.

35. When you get home, change out of your work clothes, and say hello to each of your family members, the people you live with, your pets, plants, even your couch. Take a moment to look and take five to ten minutes to be quiet and still. Wash your hands as if you are starting a new phase of your life. If you live alone, feel what it is like to enter the quietness of your environment.

Media and Resources

For further reading

- Becker, Ernest. 1971. *The Birth and Death of Meaning: An Interdisciplinary Perspective on the Problem of Man.* New York, NY: Free Press.

- Goldstein, Joseph and Jack Kornfield. 1987. *Seeking the Heart of Wisdom: The Path of Insight Meditation*. Boulder, CO: Shambhala Publications.

- Goleman, Daniel. 2003. *Destructive Emotions and How We Can Overcome Them*. New York: Bloomsbury.

- Goleman, Daniel. 2003. *Healing Emotions: Conversations with the Dalai Lama on Mindfulness, Emotions, and Health*. Boulder, CO: Shambhala Publications.

- Hạnh, Thích Nhất. 1991. *The Miracle of Mindfulness: A Manual on Meditation*. London, England: Rider Books.

- Kabat-Zinn, Jon. 1990. *Full Catastrophe Living: How to cope with Stress, Pain, and Illness Using Mindfulness Meditation*. London, England: Piatkus.

- Kabat-Zinn, Jon. 1995. *Wherever You Go, There You Are: Mindfulness Meditation for Everyday Life*. Westport, CT: Hyperion.

- Kabat-Zinn, Jon. 2005. *Coming to Our Senses: Healing Ourselves and the World Through Mindfulness*. London, England: Piatkus.

- Kabat-Zinn, Jon and Myla. 1998. *Everyday Blessings: the Inner World of Mindful Parenting*. Westport, CT: Hyperion.

- Kornfield, Jack. 1994. *A Path with Heart*. London, England: Rider Books.

- Neale, Miles Dr. 2018. *The Gradual Path: The Tibetan Buddhist Path of Becoming Fully Human*. Louisville, CO: Sounds True Publishing.

- Rosenberg, Larry. 1998. *Breath by Breath: The Liberating Practice of Insight Meditation*. London, England: Thorsons Publishing.

- Williams, Mark; John Teasdale; Zindel Segal; and Jon Kabat-Zinn. 2007. *The Mindful Way through Depression: Freeing Yourself from Chronic Unhappiness*. New York, NY: Guilford Press (includes CD of guided meditations).

Videos

- Work Mindfulness YouTube Channel
  https://www.youtube.com/channel/UCXS_IslrLrBpCVg1cJvxmMA

- 60 Minutes Mindfulness Revolution
  https://www.youtube.com/watch?v=ozyr7jVucz0

- Tara Brach – Radical Acceptance
  https://www.youtube.com/watch?v=4KIgvHntePw

Websites and other resources on mindfulness

- Center for Mindfulness in Medicine, Health Care and Society, University of Massachusetts Medical School (https://www.ummhealth.org/center-mindfulness)

- Centre for Mindfulness Research and Practice, University of Wales, Bangor, UK (www.bangor.ac.uk/mindfulness)

- Mindfulness-Based Cognitive Therapy Developments (www.mbct.com; www.mbct.co.uk)

- Oxford Cognitive Therapy Centre: (www.mbct.co.uk) follow links to mindfulness.

- Jon Kabat-Zinn guided meditations: (www.mindfulnesscds.com).

- Mindfulness is good for our bodies: A seminal study found that, after just eight weeks of training, practicing mindfulness meditation boosts the immune system's ability to fight off illness. http://www.ncbi.nlm.nih.gov/pubmed/12883106

- Mindfulness is good for our minds: Several studies have found that mindfulness increases positive emotions while reducing negative emotions and stress. Indeed, at least one study suggests it may be as good as antidepressants in fighting depression and preventing relapse.

- http://greatergood.berkeley.edu/images/uploads/Keng_Review_of_studies_on_mindfulness.pdf

- Mindfulness changes our brains: Research has found that it increases the density of gray matter in brain regions linked to learning, memory, emotion regulation, and empathy. http://greatergood.berkeley.edu/article/item/a_little_meditation_goes_a_long_way/

- Mindfulness helps us focus: Studies suggest that mindfulness helps us tune out distractions and improves our memory and attention skills.

    1. https://greatergood.berkeley.edu/article/research_digest/how_meditation_is_good_for_mind_and_body#how_mindfulness_helps_our_brains_focus

    2. https://pubmed.ncbi.nlm.nih.gov/20363650/

    3. https://pubmed.ncbi.nlm.nih.gov/22363278/

- Mindfulness fosters compassion and altruism: Research suggests mindfulness training makes us more likely to help someone in need and increases activity in neural networks involved in understanding the suffering of others and regulating emotions. Evidence suggests it might boost self-compassion as well.

    1. https://greatergood.berkeley.edu/article/item/meditation_causes_compassionate_action

    2. https://greatergood.berkeley.edu/article/item/how_to_train_the_compassionate_brain

    3. https://greatergood.berkeley.edu/article/item/does_mindfulness_make_you_compassionate

- Mindfulness enhances relationships: Research suggests mindfulness training makes couples more satisfied with their relationship, makes each partner feel more optimistic and relaxed, and makes them feel more accepting of and closer to one another. https://www.sciencedirect.com/science/article/abs/pii/S0005789404800285

- Mindfulness is good for parents and parents-to-be: Studies suggest it may reduce pregnancy-related anxiety, stress, and depression in expectant parents. Parents who practice mindfulness report being happier with their parenting skills, and their relationship with their kids, and their kids were found to have better social skills.

1. https://greatergood.berkeley.edu/article/item/ losing_my_mindfulness

2. https://greatergood.berkeley.edu/article/item/mindful_birth/

3. https://greatergood.berkeley.edu/article/item/ practice_for_parents/

- Mindfulness helps schools: There's scientific evidence that teaching mindfulness in the classroom reduces behavior problems and aggression among students, and it improves their happiness levels and ability to pay attention. Teachers trained in mindfulness also show lower blood pressure, less negative emotion and symptoms of depression, and greater compassion and empathy.

1. https://greatergood.berkeley.edu/article/item/ mindful_education

2. https://greatergood.berkeley.edu/article/item/ mindful_kids_peaceful_schools

3. https://greatergood.berkeley.edu/article/ item/a_training_to_make_teachers_less_stressed

- Mindfulness helps healthcare professionals cope with stress, connect with their patients, and improve their general quality of life. It also helps mental health professionals reduce negative emotions and anxiety and increase their positive emotions and feelings of self-compassion.

1. https://pubmed.ncbi.nlm.nih.gov/19341981/

2. https://psycnet.apa.org/record/2005-05099-004

3. https://psycnet.apa.org/record/2007-07751-003

4. https://greatergood.berkeley.edu/article/item/ try_selfcompassion/

- Mindfulness helps prisons: Evidence suggests mindfulness reduces anger, hostility, and mood disturbances among prisoners by increasing their awareness of their thoughts and emotions, helping with their rehabilitation and reintegration. https://greatergood.berkeley.edu/article/item/restorative_justice_help_prisoners_heal

- Mindfulness helps veterans: Studies suggest it can reduce the symptoms of Post-Traumatic Stress Disorder (PTSD) in the aftermath of war. https://greatergood.berkeley.edu/article/item/treating_the_wounds_of_war/

- Mindfulness fights obesity: Practicing "mindful eating" encourages healthier eating habits, helps people lose weight, and helps them savor the food they do eat. https://greatergood.berkeley.edu/article/item/better_eating_through_mindfulness

Top Five Guided Meditation Apps

- Headspace - https://www.headspace.com/
- Insight Timer - https://insighttimer.com/
- Calm - https://www.calm.com/
- The Mindfulness App - https://themindfulnessapp.com/
- Buddhify - https://buddhify.com/

Meditation Scripts

This section contains several meditation scripts that you might like to use. These scripts focus on the primary mindfulness areas of compassion, breathing, sleeping, and mindfulness during everyday activities. Use these scripts and explore the links provided in the resources section for guided meditations that you can use.

Loving-kindness meditation

Five types of people to develop loving-kindness toward:

- Yourself
- A good friend
- A "neutral" person
- A difficult person
- All four of the above equally
- And then gradually, the entire universe

Picture each of these people in your mind, and in turn, send each one loving-kindness, such as these examples below.

» *May I be well.*

» *May I be happy.*

» *May I be free from suffering.*

» *May my good friend be well.*

» *May my good friend be happy.*

» *May my good friend be free from suffering.*

» *May the neutral person I am picturing be well.*

» *May the neutral person I am picturing be happy.*

» *May the neutral person I am picturing be free from suffering.*

» *May this person I find difficult be well.*

» *May this person I find difficult be happy.*

» *May this person I find difficult be free from suffering.*

» *May all of these people including me be well.*

» *May all of these people including me be happy.*

» *May all of these people including me be free from suffering.*

» *May the entire universe be well.*

- » *May the entire universe be happy.*
- » *May the entire universe be free from suffering.*

Or

- » *May I live in safety.*
- » *May I have mental happiness (peace or joy).*
- » *May I have physical happiness (health).*
- » *May I live with ease.*
- » *May my good friend live in safety.*
- » *May my good friend have mental happiness (peace or joy).*
- » *May my good friend have physical happiness (health).*
- » *May my good friend live with ease.*
- » [Continue with each type of person.]

Or

- » *I know I (they) suffer.*
- » *Inhale the dark cloud that's around me (them).*
- » *Transform and generate the white light of compassion.* Exhale slowly three times.

[Continue with each type of person.]

Awareness of Breath Meditation

This is a guided meditation that will lead you through the process of paying attention to your breathing in every detail. It helps you get in touch with the feel of your breath and helps you practice the process of noticing when your mind wanders, bringing your attention back to your breath. This meditation improves focus and mental clarity, calms the anxious brain, and improves self-regulation.

Introduction

Awareness of breath meditation involves paying attention to the breath and will help you relax, concentrate, and improve self-awareness and your sense of well-being. It is normal for thoughts to wander, and when you lose focus and thoughts arise, other than on the breath, acknowledge it, dismiss it, and gently bring your attention back to your breath.

Find a comfortable position either sitting upright in a chair with arms and legs uncrossed or lying down with arms and legs uncrossed. You can also get in a cross-legged position or sit on the floor or on a cushion with your legs crossed. Find a place for your hands, place your palms up on your thighs with your thumb and middle finger touching.

Script

» *Start by breathing in through your nose to the count of 4 and exhaling through your mouth to the count of 8. Take a deep belly breath in through your nose to the count of 4, 1-2-3-4. Now slowly breathe out to the count of 8, pursing your lips as if you were gently blowing out a candle or blowing a bubble, 1-2-3-4-5-6-7-8. Do it again. Inhale through your nose to the count of 4, 1-2-3-4, and exhale through your mouth to the count of 8, 1-2-3-4-5-6-7-8.*

» *Now just breathe normally. As you do, notice how the air feels as it comes into your body. You might notice a feeling of the breath as it flows into your nose. Pay attention to it. Is it cool, warm, or perhaps neutral? Does it feel silky, soft, or hard? Is there an odor or fragrance?*

» *Follow the air and notice how it feels as it flows past your nostrils, up into your nasal passageways, and down the back of your throat. Notice the sensations as the air fills your lungs from the bottom, gradually filling them up to the top.*

» *Be aware of the air as you exhale. Empty your lungs starting at the top and going gradually down to the bottom. Is the air warmer as it comes up into your throat on exhalation? Observe how it feels when the air flows up your throat, into your mouth, and across your lips.*

» *Keep noticing your breath as it flows in and out of you. Send your affection and caring to this wonderful breath, as it flows down into your lungs and then back out again. Allow it to flow as it brings the life force into your being.*

» *Enjoy the feeling of nourishment and healing as you continue to breathe in and then out.*

» *Do you notice any change in your breathing now that you have been paying attention to it? Is your breathing deep? Is your breathing Shallow? Are you breathing slowly, rapidly, gently, sharply?*

» *Observe your breathing pattern without changing it. Become aware of the peace, warmth, and healing that breathing brings to your being. Allow it. Accept it. Own it. It is yours and yours alone. Allow your breath to fill every part of your body. Let it bring comfort and healing wherever it's needed.*

» *Take an intentional breath in and breathe in peace and healing. Now exhale and allow anything that needs to go to flow out effortlessly. Allow your breath to cleanse and heal. Observe it. Be with it. If your mind wanders, that's okay, accept it; every mind wanders while doing this. Just bring your attention back to your breath. Send loving thoughts to your breath.*

» *Be in touch with feelings of gratitude—be thankful for the breath that so effortlessly gives you life. Marvel at the wonder of breathing. Isn't it amazing how your body breathes automatically far beneath conscious thought? Appreciate how your body just knows what to do with this precious breath of air without any thinking or doing on your part. Just being present to what is.*

» *Take another intentional breath in through your nose to the count of 4, 1-2-3-4. Now exhale through your mouth to the count of 8, 1-2-3-4-5-6-7-8. Do it again. Inhale peace, relaxation, and harmony. Exhale and observe that what needs to go is going on its own.*

» *Now breathe normally again. Float on the cushion of your own breath. Breathing is effortless. Enjoy and appreciate the wonderful phenomenon of breathing.*

> » *Bring your awareness back to the room when you are ready.*

> » *Spend a few minutes reflecting on what came up during the meditation. Did you notice any sensations in your body? Did any particular thoughts arise? How did you handle distracting thoughts? Do they feel any different after the meditation than before doing it? Did you experience any difficulty?*

Meditation for Daily Activities

Awareness of everyday activities

A famous Zen teaching states, "Before enlightenment, chop wood and carry water; after enlightenment, chop wood and carry water." It's not very motivating for the goal-oriented practitioner! What is perhaps not immediately clear is that the quality of mind that is brought to these daily activities changes everything. Being present while chopping wood and carrying water is entirely different from mindlessly completing the same tasks.

The ultimate practice for pragmatists, applying mindfulness to daily activities involves being fully present to and mindfully aware of any one of the many daily experiences for which our minds are typically not in attendance, such as filling a glass of water or turning on the stove (the modern equivalent of the Zen classic). Therapists can help clients learn how to bring a mindful presence to any of their many routine daily tasks by quieting the mind and simply focusing on the task at hand.

Common activities include the following:

- Washing dishes
- Washing your hands
- Feeling the water in the shower or bath
- Listening to the first two rings of the phone
- Drinking the first few sips of coffee or tea in the morning
- Eating the first three bites of a meal

- Mindful sitting at a traffic light

- Feeling the breeze through a car window

- Listening to sounds from outside

- Taking a sip of water

- Smelling a flower

- Touching a fabric

Just about any experience in your day can be done mindfully. The simpler, the better.

Meditation for sleep script

» *Let's begin by doing a few deep cleansing breaths. Breathe in through your nose to the count of four and breathe out through your mouth to the count of eight. Purse your lips as you blow out, like gently blowing a bubble.*

» *Do it with me. Breathe in through your nose and then, as you exhale, relax your mind.*

» *Do it again. Breathe in relaxation and, as you breathe out, relax your mind.*

» *One more time. Breathe in comfort and, as you breathe out, let go of anything that needs to go.*

» *Now breathe normally.*

» *Pay attention to your toes. Notice how they feel. Notice if there is any tightness or discomfort there, and let it flow right out through the ends of your toes and onto the floor.*

» *Now focus on your feet: the balls of your feet, your arches, your heels, the tops of your feet. Just pay attention to what's there and let anything that needs to go flow right out through the ends of your toes and onto the floor.*

» *Now concentrate on your ankles. Just notice what they feel like. Send them loving thoughts. Allow any discomfort or tension stored there to flow down through your feet and right through to the ends of your toes and onto the floor.*

» *Now bring your awareness to your calves and shins. Again, just notice what's there. Let anything that needs to go flow right down through your ankles, your feet, and right through to the ends of your toes and onto the floor.*

» *Now bring your attention to your knees. Notice what they feel like. Let go of anything that doesn't belong. Let it flow down through your calves and shins, through your ankles, your feet, and right through to the ends of your toes and onto the floor.*

» *Now bring your awareness to your thighs. Notice what's there and allow anything that needs to go to flow down through your knees, your calves and shins, your feet, and right through to the ends of your toes and onto the floor.*

» *Now focus on your bottom. Pay attention to what you notice there. Just let go of anything that needs to go and let it flow down through your thighs, through your knees, your calves and shins, your feet, and right through to the ends of your toes and onto the floor.*

» *Now bring your attention to your lower belly or abdomen. Spend a moment to notice what you are carrying there. Allow anything that doesn't belong to flow down through your thighs, through your knees, your calves and shins, your feet, and right through to the ends of your toes and onto the floor.*

» *Now notice how your lower back feels. Lots of tension gets stored there, and you just don't need any of it. Let it flow down through your bottom, your thighs, through your knees, your calves and shins, your feet, and right through to the ends of your toes and onto the floor.*

» *Now concentrate on your stomach. Imagine that you are looking at a rope that is twisted, coiled, and tied up tightly. But as you watch the rope, it unwinds, uncoils, and unties until it is hanging limply. Imagine that your stomach and the area around your stomach have done the same and are now relaxed and comfortable.*

» *Bring your awareness to your chest and heart area. Take a nice deep breath in through your nose and fill your lungs with a cushion of healing energy. As you breathe out, allow everything to flow out that needs to go.*

» *Now pay attention to your middle and upper back. Lots of stuff gets carried there, and you don't need any of it. Allow it to flow down through your lower back, your bottom, through your thighs, through your knees, your calves and shins, your feet, and right through to the ends of your toes and onto the floor.*

» *Now focus on your neck and shoulders. Again, lots of tightness gets stored there, and you don't need it. Allow it to flow down your back, through your bottom, through your thighs, through your knees, your calves and shins, your feet, and right through to the ends of your toes and onto the floor.*

» *Now pay attention to your hands including your fingers, thumbs, palms, and backs of your hands. Notice what you carry there, and let go of anything you don't need. Let it flow through to the ends of your fingers and onto the floor.*

» *Now pay attention to your arms including your forearms, elbows, and upper arms right up to your shoulders. Let anything you don't need flow down through your arms, your wrists, your hands, and right through to the ends of your fingers and onto the floor.*

» *Now raise your awareness to your face including your jaw, cheeks, eyes, and forehead. Drop your jaw and just let it hang totally limp. Let any tension stored in your face flow down through your neck, shoulders, arms, hands, and right through to the ends of your fingers and onto the floor.*

» *Now pay attention to your brain. As thoughts arise, imagine they are written on a blank whiteboard. As soon as you see them there, erase them and imagine the board is empty again.*

» *Now that your body is completely relaxed and starting to doze, imagine that you are walking along a path in the forest. Take a slow deep breath. The air smells so fresh here, so clean and natural. You feel connected to the earth. You can hear the birds singing. You notice how the sun is shining down through the leaves and creating beautiful sunlight-and-shadow patterns on the forest floor. The forest floor itself is lush and green. You feel so happy, alive, and content.*

» *As you walk along, you gradually reach the edge of the forest and walk into a beautiful meadow. The air is clear, the sun is shining, the sky is blue, and the temperature is just perfect. You can see pretty butterflies and beautiful flowers all around you. You notice the path here is worn smooth from many feet, so you sit down and take off your shoes and socks. You walk along the path barefoot, and you feel the smooth, warm earth on the bottoms of your feet. You feel connected to the earth, nature, and infinite intelligence.*

» *The path starts to become sandy, and you realize you are walking toward a beautiful lake. You can smell the freshness of the water and the wet sand. The water on the lake is so calm it looks like a mirror. You can see the trees perfectly reflected in the lake around the edges. The sky is blue, and the air feels fresh and clean. You can see some flowers blooming at the edge of the beach and some lilies growing on the shore. Listen carefully. You can hear the water as it gently laps up against the shore. Mmm… it feels good here, so peaceful, so safe. If you feel like it, walk along the edge of the water and feel the cool, clear water on your feet.*

» *As you walk, you look ahead on the beach and see a chaise lounge sitting on the sand. You walk over to it and lie down on it. Its cushions are soft and feel so comfortable when you lie down. You notice a blanket underneath and you reach down to get it and cover yourself. You snuggle down.*

» *As you lie on the chaise, you let your mind slow down some more. You let go, and any busy thoughts disappear as you tell your monkey brain to calm down and relax. You feel warm and cozy. As you take some slow deep breaths, you begin to feel warm and heavy all over your body. Your eyelids get so heavy you can't keep them open anymore. Allow them to close. Listen to my voice as you let go of your day and begin to drift and allow sleep to come to you.*

» *You realize you are in your own comfortable bed. You are safe. You feel so comfortable and relaxed. You fall into a deep, restful sleep. You sleep soundly all night. You will awake in the morning exactly when you need to be awake to start your day, and you will feel completely rested, rejuvenated, and wide-awake. You will have the right amount of energy and you feel happy.*

» *You will look forward to your day. You will notice you are completely focused, and you can concentrate effortlessly. You will know what you need to do, and you will get everything done you need to do. You will be on time. You will get along with everyone, and your friends and family will be happy to see you. You will stay focused, calm, relaxed, and happy all day. You know you will sleep well again at night.*

» *Sleeping is easy now. Allow your brain to let go. Allow sleep to arrive. Sleep is here now. Sleep, sleep, sleep. Goodnight.*

Afterword

Thank you for reading The Mindfulness Experience. I really hope you enjoyed the book, and we can continue to keep in touch.

I invite you to go to my website at www.workmindfulness.com, to join our community. Or join our Facebook group at the link below: https://www.facebook.com/groups/themindfulnessexperience

Most importantly, if the book has helped you, please recommend it to others. If you have a minute to spare, I would be very grateful if you could write a short review on the page or site where you bought the book. Your help in spreading the word is greatly appreciated. Reviews from readers like you make a huge difference to helping new readers find ways to improve their lives through more mindful experiences.

Thank you!

Keith W Fiveson
Email: kfiveson@workmindfulness.com
Twitter: https://twitter.com/kfiveson

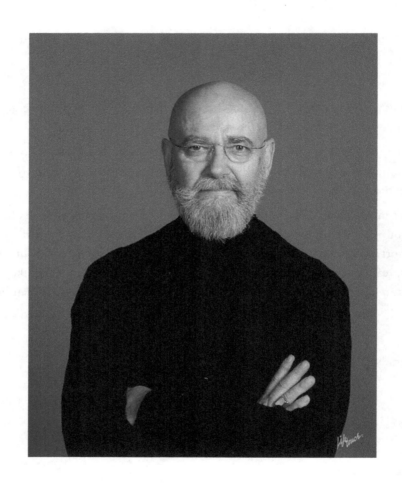

About the Author

KEITH W FIVESON is a sixty-five-year-old yogi who has studied life in all its challenges. For the past thirty years, his mission has been to help individuals and organizations become more conscious, awake, and alive to life and all its opportunities. With this book, *The Mindfulness Experience*, he has distilled the wisdom of the ages. As a survivor and thriver, he has built a life of presence, to be aware of every sacred moment of truth. He overcame cancer twice, a heart condition, a broken home, challenging relationships, and a childhood family life that was dysfunctional and abusive.

Keith has traveled extensively, working and studying, in over forty-five countries worldwide. He is a certified life coach, Thai yoga therapist, and meditation teacher. He has practiced and studied Eastern and Western mindfulness/meditation for over twenty-five years. He started to cultivate his practice over thirty years ago, using his army training to balance a very hectic corporate career. He has extensive experience in the corporate world, working under extreme pressure and stress with incredible people and companies.

Keith is an alumnus of Price Waterhouse Coopers and the founder of IT Enabled Services Alliance, Inc., a global consulting firm. He has held executive positions at British Telecom, AT&T, and MCI Telecommunications, later to become Verizon Business. Back in the early days of the internet, he helped develop solutions for Best Buy, CUNA, Apple, McGraw-Hill, Time Warner, Autism Speaks, General Electric, Citibank, and Merrill Lynch, among others.

He lives in Port Washington, NY, and he works actively in several communities. He coaches several high-functioning executives and individuals who wish to live their best life now, with balance, in an unbalanced world.